Treating Thyroid Disease Symptoms, Problems and Complications

A Compilation of Thyroid Book Titles

By: James M. Lowrance © 2012

INTRODUCTION:

This ebook is a compilation of thyroid disease titles I have written (43 Chapters and 87 "Q & As" -- approx. 71,582 words in length), that cover the subjects of problematic hypothyroid and hyperthyroid symptomology and how these are treated. People with disorders affecting their thyroid glands, often experience a variety of different problem-symptoms and complications, that are not always resolved by their initial medical treatments.

In these cases, specialized attention by their treating doctors is required and in most cases more diligence on the part of the patients is required as well. It is my hope that this book of compiled titles I have written regarding the more complicated thyroid disease symptoms, serves to provide a worthy educational resource for those who read it.

3

TABLE OF CONTENTS:

(NOTE: Some lifestyle practices information regarding goitrogen foods, supplements and diet discussed in this section are repeated from "SECTION TWO" regarding thyroid cancer)

(NOTE: The "Spirituality" aspect in this section, is in reference to fundamental Christian views.)

4

SECTION ONE:

Antibodies that Cause Thyroid Diseases and Symptoms

(Immune Cells causing Hypothyroidism & Hyperthyroidism)

5

TABLE OF CONTENTS:

CHAPTER ONE

Facts about Thyroid Antibodies

The majority of patients with both hypothyroidism (under-active thyroid) and hyperthyroidism (overactive thyroid) are experiencing autoimmune diseases that cause these conditions. When autoimmune thyroid disease results in hypothyroidism, the term for the disease is "Hashimoto's thyroiditis." When the autoimmune disease of the thyroid causes hyperthyroidism, it is called "Grave's Disease."

Thyroid antibodies attack key proteins in the thyroid gland and in some cases, stimulate production of excessive amounts of hormone. These killer cells that are manufactured by the immune system become confused for reasons yet to be fully understood by medical science and they begin to identify thyroid cells as threats in the body. As they attack these cells, the thyroid gland becomes damaged, resulting in inflammation, enlargement of the gland (goiter) and thyroid hormone imbalances.

Protein-Enzyme Cell Destroying Antibodies

The antibodies, also called "auto-antibodies", that enter into thyroid protein-enzymes, causing destruction of them, are called the "Anti-thyroidperoxidase" and the "Anti-thyroglobulin". Abbreviations commonly used for these on medical blood lab documents are "TPO ABs" and "TG ABs" or "Anti-TPO" and "Anti-TG".

Once these proteins called thyroidperoxidase and thyroglobulin are destroyed by these antibodies, they are rendered incapable of aiding in the process of converting iodine absorbed by the thyroid gland, into thyroid hormones that regulate the metabolism of all other cells in the body. This is the rate at which the body burns fuels that enter the body, converting them into energy.

As fewer hormones become available the metabolism can be slowed down (hypothyroidism). These proteins are also part of what keeps thyroid tissue healthy and so as the level of them begins to diminish, thyroid tissue will also begin to die within the gland. As this process occurs, the thyroid gland can become inflamed (thyroiditis) and/or enlarged (goiter).

Thyroid Stimulating Antibodies

These antibodies are also called "Thyroid Stimulating Immunoglobulin" (abbreviated TSI). These type auto-antibodies stimulate excessive release of T3-triiodothyronine and T4-thyroxine from the thyroid gland. They do this by binding to receptors in the blood that normally attach to the Thyroid Stimulating Hormone (TSH) which is another hormone that comes from the pituitary brain-gland that regulates hormone release from the thyroid gland.

TSH in-essence is a messenger hormone, telling the thyroid gland how much hormone is needed in the body and keeps the levels in-balance for proper metabolism via ongoing communication.

Once the TSI antibodies attach to TSH-receptors, the message from them to the thyroid gland mimics the communication of TSH which stimulates an increase in thyroid hormone levels. They are in-essence tricking the thyroid gland into producing more thyroid hormone when it is not needed, causing a sped up metabolism in the body (hyperthyroidism).

Graves' Disease and Hashimoto's Thyroiditis

All three types of antibodies described in the previous subheadings can be present in both Graves' disease and Hashimoto's thyroiditis. Graves', results in eventual hyperthyroidism in most cases and Hashimoto's results in hypothyroidism. The diseases are differentiated and diagnosed by the balance of auto-antibodies found, by levels of thyroid hormones in the body (imbalances) and by the symptom manifestations caused by the combination of these two factors.

The TPO and TG antibodies are typically found in higher titers (lab measurements) in Hashimoto's patients than in Graves' patients, so both diseases cause thyroid gland destruction but at a much slower rate with Graves' disease. The TSI antibodies that stimulate excessive hormone release from the thyroid gland are found to be high-positive in the vast majority of Graves' patients but are not found to be positive in all Hashimoto's patients and when they are, it is usually in low titers. If a Hashimoto's patient does have significant levels of TSI, it can cause, intermittent phases of hyperthyroidism, called "Hashitoxicosis" which is most often a temporary condition.

These facts about antibodies point to how closely related Graves' and Hashimoto's are and may also explain as to why patients with one disease may transition over to the other in rare cases when a significant change in the balance of auto-antibodies and thyroid hormone levels takes place.

The five subheadings below help to bring better understanding to the subject of "thyroid antibodies."

Thyroid antibodies cause "autoimmune thyroid disease" in patients who develop them.

The immune system normally sends out antibodies, which are killer cells, to eradicate foreign invaders from the body that can make us sick. These invaders include viruses, bacteria and allergens. The purpose of antibodies is to seek these out and destroy them, so as to prevent our bodies from becoming ill. The problem with "thyroid antibodies" is that, like other antibodies that cause autoimmune diseases, they are directed against the thyroid gland as if it is one of these invaders. It is a case of mistaken identity that over time causes damage to the thyroid gland and cell death. Eventually, the antibodies will kill out the thyroid gland completely (hypothyroidism).

Some thyroid antibodies cause hypothyroidism, while others cause hyperthyroidism.

The two autoimmune diseases caused by thyroid antibodies are "Hashimoto's Disease (thyroiditis), which results in hypothyroidism, and "Grave's Disease", which results in hyperthyroidism.

The types that cause Hashimoto's Disease relentlessly attack the thyroid, until it becomes damaged and unable to function at its original level. Once enough damage has been done to the gland and a significant percent of thyroid cells have been killed, the onset of hypothyroidism occurs. The low level of functioning will usually be mild at first (sub-clinical) and over time will worsen, unless the patient with hypothyroidism receives treatment. The opposite is true of patients with Grave's Disease because in their case, the antibodies directed against the thyroid gland stimulate it to produce excessive amounts of thyroid hormone or a high functioning thyroid gland.

What are the main antibodies tested for in these two types of autoimmune thyroid diseases?

In Hashimoto's Disease, the two main antibodies that cause thyroid gland destruction and resulting hypothyroidism are the anti-Thyroid Peroxidase Antibodies (abbreviated TPO) and the anti-Thyroglobulin Antibodies (abbreviated TG). In Grave's Disease, the main antibody that causes stimulation of the thyroid gland to produce too much hormone is called the Thyroid Stimulating Immunoglobulin (abbreviated TSI). The antibodies for both diseases types of diseases are detected by means of blood lab tests.

What are the symptoms that prompt testing for thyroid antibodies that, cause hypothyroidism?

The following symptoms prompt testing for thyroid antibodies that cause an under active thyroid gland:

- increased sensitivity to cold
- constipation
- dry skin
- puffy face
- hoarse voice
- elevated blood cholesterol
- unexplained weight gain
- joint aches, tenderness and stiffness
- muscle pain and weakness
- heavier than normal menstrual periods
- fatigue
- enlarged thyroid gland (goiter)
- depression

These symptoms may prompt a doctor to orders tests for the antibodies that cause Hashimoto's thyroiditis, also referred to as "chronic lymphocytic thyroiditis".

What symptoms prompt testing for thyroid antibodies that cause hyperthyroidism (overactive thyroid)?

The following symptoms prompt testing for thyroid antibodies that cause hyperthyroidism.

- sudden weight loss, even if appetite and food intake remains normal or increases
- rapid heartbeat (tachycardia - more than 100 beats a minute)
- irregular heartbeat (arrhythmia/palpitations)
- nervousness, anxiety or anxiety attacks
- irritability
- tremor (fine trembling in your hands and fingers)
- sweating ---

- changes in menstrual patterns
- increased sensitivity to heat
- changes in bowel patterns (frequent bowel movements)
- enlarged thyroid gland - goiter (swelling at the front-base of the neck)
- fatigue
- muscle weakness
- difficulty sleeping

If one or more of these symptoms are being experienced, this may prompt a doctor to orders tests for the antibodies that cause Grave's Disease, also referred to as "toxic diffuse goiter".

Thyroid diseases can develop at any age but the most common age of onset is between 35 and 40 years of age. It is recommended that adults be tested for thyroid disease at age 35 but they should be tested at any age that symptoms indicating thyroid disease may develop. Thyroid diseases affect women more commonly than men (from 5 to 8 times more often in females). Pregnancy increases the risk for the onset of thyroid disease and so pregnant women need to have their thyroid function tested as well.

Possible Triggers for Thyroid Autoimmunity

Viruses - Some medical research conclusions have cited the Epstein-Barr virus (EBV) as a possible cause of autoimmune thyroid disease. The research studies state that patients with autoimmune thyroiditis tested positive for blood levels of EBV antigens, significantly more often in the thyroid disease group than in the healthy control group.

While EBV was the virus studied, there are a number of possible viruses that can trigger autoimmune diseases in susceptible individuals. Many of these viruses, especially those in the herpes family, are contracted in early life and carried life-long. It may be that the immune system's failure to fully eradicate the body of these viruses causes it to begin attacking organs or tissues in the body that contain the virus, including the thyroid gland. Some patients, who develop sub-acute thyroiditis (temporary) that is often triggered by respiratory viruses, go on to develop permanent autoimmune thyroiditis. It may be that these individuals were predisposed to develop thyroid disease once exposed to any number of possible triggers.

Environmental Toxins - Research studies on possible causes of thyroid autoimmunity have also proposed the possibility of environmental toxins as being a common cause for the immune system attacking the thyroid gland. As the body accumulates these toxins, which the body recognizes as allergens or as strong intolerances, the immune system is triggered in trying to control these things that are in-essence acting as poisons in the body. Elevated levels of radioactivity (ionizing radiation), such as may be experienced by those who work at nuclear power facilities or at x-ray imaging labs that are over-exposed or not properly protected, can develop autoimmune thyroid diseases. This type of toxin has been well-substantiated as a cause, including studies of children exposed to radiation following the 1986 Chernobyl nuclear power plant accident in Ukraine that caused radioactive fallout. A significant number of children and young adults tested positive for thyroid antibodies in studies conducted 6 to 8 years following the accident.

Other toxins and pollutants that have been studied and that are considered strong possibilities for causing thyroid autoimmunity include toxins found in our water systems, additives and preservatives found in manufactured foods and excessive exposure to fluoride.

Stress - Chronic stress has been studied in relation to many diseases and proposed as a cause for them. This includes inflammatory and autoimmune diseases, types of cancers and immune deficiency illnesses including Chronic Fatigue Syndrome and Fibromyaligia. Many thyroid patients report that they experienced a severe or prolonged period of stress (chronic) just before the onset of their autoimmune thyroid diseases. This association has been better substantiated in patients studied who have Graves' disease, the autoimmune-caused hyperthyroid condition. While less, studies cite stress as a factor in Hashimoto's thyroiditis patients, it would seem obvious that a triggered autoimmune response can result in either condition because all types of thyroid auto-antibodies can be found in both types of thyroid diseases.

CHAPTER TWO

Do Thyroid Antibodies Cause Symptoms Apart From Abnormal Hormone Levels?

I have corresponded with many fellow autoimmune hypothyroid patients since the year 2003 and have read the testimonies of hundreds of others, in articles and on forums and message boards. What I hear from these patients, is something I have found to be true in my own case as an autoimmune hypothyroid patient (Hashimoto's Disease) and that is the fact that we can continue to experience mild to moderate symptoms, even while on optimal "thyroid hormone replacement medication" treatment. These symptoms can be intermittent or with some patients continual. The more fortunate patients rarely have symptoms while on treatment.

Surveys of thyroid patients on treatment have been conducted, the majority of the patients studied, being on the recommended optimal dose of thyroid hormone replacement medications and many taking natural T-4 and T-3 combination medications. The surveys had the respondents to report the effectiveness of their treatments and the results released in these studies, concluded that a majority of patients continued to experience a degree of symptoms. As I continued to research this subject online, I found research articles by reputable medical research groups, stating that the disease process itself, caused by thyroid antibodies - TPO (thyroid peroxidase antibodies) and the TG (thyroglobulin antibodies), can also be a factor in causing symptoms.

These research articles concluded that elevated levels of these antibodies can cause fibromyalgia type symptoms for example, in persons with only sub-clinical hypothyroidism. Other medical research articles state that autoimmune thyroid disease can also have a degree of systemic (system-wide) effect, so that the immune system response affects not only the thyroid gland but other parts of the body as well.

Here is a one-sentence quote from one of those sources:

"However, a responsibility of the mechanisms involved in the autoimmunity rather than a direct action of thyroid hormones seems supported by the evidences that some rheumatic manifestations may occur even in euthyroid patients, or that they are more frequent in hypothyroid patient with autoimmune thyroiditis than in those without this disease."

(PubMed – Title: "Chronic autoimmune thyroiditis and rheumatic manifestations." – Quotes/Reprints are allowed for public education.)

This research article and many others, clearly attribute thyroid antibody levels to symptoms, apart from thyroid hormone levels.

CHAPTER THREE

Hereditary Autoimmune Thyroid Disease

Recently on a Thyroid Health forum I was moderating, a member asked about hereditary autoimmune thyroid disease and what their chances were, as the child of a thyroid disease parent, for eventually experiencing the onset of the disease. Following bellow was my response to that question.

According to Dr. Hossein Gharib, M.D. of the American Association of Clinical Endocrinologists (AACE) and Professor at the Mayo Medical School, "Fifty percent of thyroid disease patients' offspring will inherit the thyroid disease gene."

I actually didn't know that chances for children of thyroid disease parents were at 50% risk until I found that quote from the MD above. I knew it was a high percent risk but 50% was surprising. That's not great news for children of thyroid disease parents but shows the importance of getting blood tested at any point thyroid type symptoms may arise for both the presence of thyroid antibodies and abnormal thyroid hormone levels and if symptoms don't manifest earlier, to start getting tested at age 35 regardless.

Some reputable thyroid statistics state that between ages 35 and 40 is a common age for the onset of thyroid disease. If you are the child of a parent or parents with thyroid disease, you should educate yourself about thyroid disease symptoms, so that you can recognize when there is a need to be tested, before age 35.

In my opinion, when symptoms arise in someone at risk for developing thyroid disease, they should have not only tests ordered for thyroid function but also the ones to detect "thyroid antibodies". These are the killer cells mentioned earlier that the immune system creates and sends out to attack what it perceives as invaders in the body (i.e. viruses & allergens). In the case of autoimmune thyroid disease, it recognizes the thyroid as one of those invaders. These antibodies can cause thyroid disease symptoms in advance of causing eventual thyroid hormone imbalance and is why I believe they are important to have tested in addition to thyroid hormone levels.

To repeat, the thyroid antibodies that should be tested for are the "anti-thyroidperoxidase" (TPO),"anti-thyroglobulin" (TG) and "thyroid stimulating imunnoglobulin" (TSI). Those first two are common findings (found to be positive) in autoimmune hypothyroidism or "Hashimoto's thyroiditis", while that third one is more commonly found in people with autoimmune hyperthyroidism or Grave's Disease, so depending upon the symptoms one is having, they may want only certain ones tested for.

The thyroid function tests, that detect thyroid hormone imbalances in the blood, are the "TSH" (Thyroid Stimulating Hormone), "T-4" (thyroxine) and "T-3" (triiodothyronine) levels. Some Doctors believe the "free" levels of the T-4 and T-3 are best, as opposed to the "total" levels and from what I've read in regard to their research on the subject, I happen to agree with them.

These are the ones I have tested in follow-up on my own thyroid hormone therapy for hypothyroidism but are also good tests for diagnosing thyroid disorders as well. If only one test is used to evaluate thyroid function, it will usually be the TSH level. This one is the pituitary hormone that accurately reflects how well the thyroid gland is supplying hormone to the body and is sensitive in that it usually detects a change in thyroid function earlier than any other blood test.

CHAPTER FOUR

Epstein-Barr Virus a Cause of Autoimmune Thyroid Disease?

There is medical research that has been published in regard to the Epstein-Barr Virus (EBV) and its role in causing autoimmune thyroiditis and other autoimmune and neurological diseases. It is also highly associated with contributing to the development of different types of cancer. I believe that EBV may be the cause of my own Hashimoto's thyroiditis and the resulting hypothyroidism (under-active thyroid) I began to experience at age 39. I suffered a severe case of mononucleosis at approximately 10 years of age that I highly suspect to have negatively affected my immune system.

Thyroid disease, especially the autoimmune type runs in families, in fact children of one parent that has thyroid disease, has a 50% chance of also developing thyroid disease during their lifetime. As mentioned earlier, Hossein Gharib, M.D., F.A.C.E, president-elect of AACE and Professor of Medicine at the Mayo Medical School states that "Fifty percent of thyroid disease patients' offspring will inherit the thyroid disease gene."

When I personally was diagnosed with thyroid hormone imbalance and later diagnosed with Hashimoto's Autoimmune Thyroiditis, I naturally wondered what caused me to have susceptibility to this disease. I knew that thyroid diseases were experienced far more often in women than in men.

My mother however does not have thyroid autoimmunity but did develop age related hypothyroidism, common in women over the age of 60. I also knew my dad does not have thyroid disease or any other type of autoimmune disease. This is what led me to reflect on any childhood diseases that might have triggered the later-life autoimmune thyroid disease I am now experiencing.

When looking back at my childhood, I realized that I developed the severe case of mononucleosis at age 10. This is the disease caused by EBV (also called "the kissing disease") and after contracting it, the virus remains in your body lifelong. While my siblings (one sister and two brothers), may very well have been exposed to the virus and are now lifelong carriers, they did not experience mono as I did. My mono symptoms were the typical ones, including severely swollen lymph glands in my neck, fever and severe fatigue. In fact, I was taken out of school due to the case of mono, for about six weeks.

My belief is that the virus causing mono in my childhood compromised my immune system and left me vulnerable to developing Hashimoto's thyroiditis as an adult, which also involves the lymphatic system. Another name for Hashimoto's is Chronic Lymphocytic Thyroiditis.

I feel it is possible that as the research articles about EBV and autoimmune thyroiditis point out, EBV will cause the immune system over time, to attack tissues in the body that are infiltrated with the virus via antibodies it creates in attempt to eradicate it from the body.

The immune system is relentless and if it cannot eradicate a virus over time, it may then begin to attack the tissues in the body that contain the virus (autoimmunity). In the case of autoimmune thyroid disease, the immune system creates the TPO, TG and TSI antibodies that replicate to high numbers, to eradicate this mistakenly perceived enemy of the body – the thyroid gland.

When I was rechecked for EBV levels in my blood, shortly following my diagnosis of thyroid disease, I had very high titers of the virus still in my system, as reflected by the antibody levels that correlate with the virus levels. My result on the blood lab test for EBV antibodies (reflecting the level of virus they are attacking) was "218" with normal values being less that "20". My elevations of the virus were more that 10 times the normal range. While I will never be able to prove with certainty that EBV caused my autoimmune thyroid disease, I will always highly suspect that it is indeed the cause in my case.

CHAPTER FIVE

Hashimoto's Encephalopathy Rare but Serious

There is a neuro-endocrine disorder that causes very serious and potentially life threatening symptoms, called Hashimoto's Encephalopathy (HE). The disorder can occur in patients with Hashimoto's thyroiditis, who experience a very high elevation of "thyroid antibody" levels. These antibodies, that attack the thyroid gland after recognition of it by the immune system, as a foreign invader, can become highly elevated in these rare cases of HE. At these high elevations they will begin to affect brain and nerve function in the body or the "neurological system". Severe symptoms will result because this system is the body's information and communication center and a disruption from a disease process can cause an array of nerve and brain related symptoms.

Inflammation caused by the antibodies (also called auto-antibodies) spreads to the brain and begins to affect the tissue containing the nerves that control bodily functions and impulses throughout the body. The resulting effects are severe neurological symptoms, meaning abnormal responses and manifestations of nervous system dysfunction. These symptoms can include the following.

• psychotic episodes (hallucinations and delusions)
• dementia (mental deterioration)
• neuropathies (abnormal nerve sensations)
• seizures
• coma
• possible death if left untreated.

The antibodies responsible for causing thyroid destruction and inflammation in the thyroid gland but that can rarely also result in HE when highly elevated, are the "TPO" (anti-thyroidperoxidase) and "TG" (anti-thyroglobulin) antibodies. The less common manifestation of chronic lymphocytic thyroiditis, called Hashimoto's Encephalopathy, is more often a result of elevated anti-TPO levels although it can result from elevations of both it and the anti-TG antibodies in some cases.

Thyroid hormone levels are not usually a factor in this potentially serious neuro-endocrine disorder of thyroid autoimmunity. Some patients in fact have been documented in medical research, to have experienced HE with their thyroid hormone levels in normal range and before they were in need of thyroid hormone replacement therapy. This disorder is a rare but strong example of the fact that thyroid antibodies have the ability to produce bodily symptoms regardless of thyroid hormone levels.

Treatment for HE, is to reduce the inflammation caused by the thyroid antibodies by administering a steroid anti-inflammatory drug to patients who are diagnosed. These drugs, also called corticosteroids or hydrocortisone, mimic the anti-inflammatory properties of our body's own natural anti-inflammatory called "cortisol". A major brand prescribed for inflammatory conditions is "Prednisone", a powerful steroid that usually achieves an anti-inflammatory effect quickly with only a relatively short term regimen being necessary to correct cases of HE. Patients, who are treated, usually see a complete reversal of symptoms and will not experience any long term complications from HE, once it has been resolved with treatment.

25

If a patient with Hashimoto's thyroiditis or their loved ones, notice the onset of sudden and severe neurological symptoms, they should report to their Doctor immediately, to rule out HE as the cause. A delay in treatment for a patient experiencing this very rare disorder could result in severe consequences.

CHAPTER SIX

My Own Experience with Thyroid Antibody Related Symptoms

Sometime ago, I had an office visit with an Endocrinologist and I took my LabOne blood test results with me. He found on the results, that my thyroid hormone levels were at optimal range (free T-3 was at top of normal) but even though I had been on hormone replacement medication (Armour), for over two years to treat hypothyroidism, my TG and TPO antibodies were still elevated. My TG ABs, were "537" (normal range <40), so were about 500 points above normal. My TPO ABs, were "120" (normal range <35), so were about 85 points above normal.

My complaint at that time was continuing mild to moderate joint pain, especially in my upper spine and shoulders and moderate, intermittent fatigue. His response to this was that elevated antibody levels also mean there is resulting "inflammation" and that this could cause these symptoms, apart from my normal thyroid hormone levels. I was amazed that other Doctors I had seen and even the drug manufacturer's websites, did not mention the role of thyroid antibodies, in causing ongoing symptoms, despite proper thyroid hormone replacement therapy.

My Endocrinologist prescribed me a short-term round of "corticosteroids" (anti-inflammatory steroid) and told me afterward that I could take occasional over-the-counter anti-inflammatory medications such as Ibuprofen to help with any intermittent symptom-flares.

Since that time, my joint pain has diminished to only rare, mild occurrence and I rarely have the need to take an anti-inflammatory for rheumatic (joint and muscle) symptoms but I do still have occasional bouts of mild to moderate fatigue. Occasionally I suffer severe flares of fatigue if I experience chronic stress or if I allow stimulants in my diet that I have sensitivities to (i.e. caffeine, chocolate and alcohol).

I am not sure why more is not being stated in regard to this area of the role thyroid antibodies have in causing symptoms because it makes complete sense that highly activated immune system activity, can result in a bodily response manifesting in different degrees of symptoms, depending upon how highly elevated antibody and resulting inflammation levels are. Inflammation from the autoimmune disease process also manifests in symptoms, which means the disease process itself is also what also causes the illness and not the resulting hypothyroidism alone.

When patients complain to their Doctors about symptoms but their hormone levels are replaced to optimal levels, the Doctor may tell the patient that their symptoms cannot be thyroid disease related because their hormone levels have been corrected. I have heard this scenario related by many patients in correspondence with them however, when these patients ask for a retest of their thyroid antibodies levels, and they will often come back highly elevated. I have heard some patients report TPO levels in the 1,000s which would seem to be a prime candidate for explaining symptom flares they are experiencing but some Doctors seem to believe the antibody levels are insignificant in relation to symptoms.

28

It is the opinion of much medical research that has been conducted, that thyroid antibodies do indeed play a direct role in thyroid disease symptoms, apart from thyroid hormone levels and it is my I hope that continued medical research and surveys will be conducted in this area.

CHAPTER SEVEN

Autoimmune Hypothyroidism (Hashimoto's) a Cause of Chronic Fatigue Syndrome

While searching for new thyroid disease related information on the web, I came across a medical research article first published in the "Townsend Letter for Doctors and Patents" and re-printed by Dr. Alan R. Gaby M.D. The article reports findings in regard to patients with "chronic fatigue", stating that a large percent of them were found in a medical study, to have the type of lymphocytic thyroiditis that causes hypothyroidism (Hashimoto's thyroiditis). The article is entitled; "Autoimmune thyroiditis as a cause of chronic fatigue".

The interesting aspect of this report is the fact that these patients were not found to have abnormal (outside of normal values) thyroid hormone levels but despite this fact, were suffering symptoms of hypothyroidism. The autoimmune type of thyroiditis they were suffering from, that was causing the chronic fatigue, was instead diagnosed through a thyroid tissue biopsy called "Fine Needle Aspiration". This is a procedure in which a hypodermic needle is inserted into the thyroid gland and a small sample of the gland is extracted to be analyzed for the presence of diseased thyroid tissue cells.

What is important about this article, is the fact that hypothyroidism does not have to be present, for autoimmune thyroiditis to cause symptoms. In this case, the research study confirms that the symptom of chronic fatigue is one of those that can potentially be experienced, before thyroid hormone levels become abnormal.

This study is one of many that confirm the development of symptoms from thyroid autoimmunity, in advance of hypothyroidism, that is not yet detectable through blood testing of the hormone levels. Other medical research articles on the subject of hypothyroid symptoms caused by the thyroid disease process itself, apart from hormone levels, include the development of rheumatic and fibromyalgic type symptoms as mentioned in a previous chapter.

In addition to my finding these articles and other research for my own articles, through online searching, these past several years, I have also corresponded with many thyroid disease patients attesting to having developed hypothyroid symptoms from thyroid autoimmunity, in advance of their thyroid hormone levels becoming abnormal as detected by blood lab test results. Despite all of the information that is available out there on this subject and reported by the most reputable medical research entities that exist, there are still Doctors treating thyroid disorders, who do not believe symptoms can develop in patients with autoimmune thyroid disease, before thyroid hormone levels fall outside of normal values.

In my own case of being diagnosed with autoimmune thyroid disease - Hashimoto's thyroiditis, also referred to as chronic lymphocytic thyroiditis, I did have abnormal hormone levels on my thyroid panel (i.e. elevated TSH and a low T-3 Uptake), in addition to testing positive for the thyroid antibodies (auto-antibodies) that cause the disease. My hormone levels were not greatly abnormal but the symptoms I was experiencing, including chronic fatigue were severe despite my hypothyroidism not being considered "full-blown" (overt) at that point.

Even if there were no research articles stating these facts, in my opinion, it is simply common sense to recognize that the disease process itself has symptom-producing potential. It is after-all autoimmune disease we are talking about and all diseases with autoimmunity as the cause result in inflammation and destruction of tissues in the body that are affected. To think that this type disease process only causes symptoms when it affects hormone levels in the body, takes much of the attention away from the seriousness of the disease process that eventually results in the abnormal hormone levels. Chronic fatigue can obviously be one of the early symptoms of an autoimmune disease process in the body, including that which affects the thyroid gland.

CHAPTER EIGHT

Doctors Should Test for Thyroid Antibodies

Better qualified Endocrinologists, Thyroid Specialists and other types of MDs who treat thyroid disorders, believe in testing for thyroid antibodies.

Sometime ago, I was corresponding with a lady, whose husband was suffering symptoms that matched those listed for thyroid disorder, specifically those of "hyperthyroidism" (i.e. anxiety, insomnia, weight loss, excessive energy, fatigue etc...). Her husband was tested for his TSH and thyroid hormone levels and the results were within the normal ranges however, the man's TSH was on the increase (his result was above 3.5). According to the new, revised TSH lab standards, set by the AACE (American Association of Clinical Endocrinologists) in the year 2002, this is not a normal TSH level. The new range set by the AACE for TSH is "0.3 to 3.0" (readings above 3.0 are suspect for hypothyroidism). In my discussion with this woman, who was seeking help on behalf of her husband, I told her that her husband's TSH would merit a test of "thyroid antibodies".

Following was my reply:

"A TSH of 3.58 is not as normal as some Doctors would have you believe. The AACE which is the organization that sets the standard for thyroid testing and treatment, released a new, revised TSH range in late 2002, having "3.0" as the cut off for high normal TSH.

Here's a quote from the AACE:

"Now the AACE encourages physicians to consider treatment for patients who test outside the boundaries of a narrower margin based on a target TSH level of 0.3 to 3.0." (The AACE)

The National Institutes of Health website actually states that a person testing with a TSH of above 2.0, should be monitored closely for development of thyroid disease.

Here is a quote from the NIH:

"Some people with a TSH value over 2.0 mIU/L, who have no signs or symptoms suggestive of an under-active thyroid, may develop hypothyroidism sometime in the future." (NIH/NLM - MedLinePlus.com, reprints allowed for public education.)

My suggestion to you is to find a qualified thyroid-treating Doctor and to have your husband tested for thyroid antibodies. These can reveal the presence of thyroid disease, in patients with normal-ish hormone levels. The tests are for the "TPO, TG and TSI" antibodies and a positive reading on one or more of these indicate thyroid autoimmunity. People with developing autoimmune hypothyroidism (Hashimoto's thyroiditis) for example, can have elevated antibody levels that cause symptoms, even with hormones being within normal-range. Patients with Hashimoto's thyroiditis (most common cause of hypothyroidism), can experience a period of hyperthyroidism, before the onset of hypothyroidism begins and progresses and the term for this is "Hashitoxicosis".

Here is a quote from a page on the WiKi website:

"Hashitoxicosis is an autoimmune thyroid disorder, in which individuals with autoimmune hypothyroidism, usually Hashimoto's thyroiditis (HT), experience intermittent or sporadic periods where they also have symptoms of hyperthyroidism." (Graves Disease and Hyperthyroidism - WikiWebsite Page)

Amazingly, some Doctors will argue these points, despite the fact that the most reputable medical sources available are stating them. Some Doctors believe and state that antibody testing is not necessary unless hormone levels fall outside of the normal reference ranges but the fact is that autoimmune thyroid disease is usually present long before it affects the hormone levels.

This would be my suggestion; to get him tested for "thyroid antibodies". It may confirm or rule out thyroid disease but will be difficult to move on to other possible causes of symptoms, if they are not tested for.

Some Doctors jump to snap-diagnoses of emotional problems, such as anxiety and depression, before ordering more complete blood evaluation for patients with both mental and physical symptoms and in my opinion, this is a disservice to them. I believe people with multi-symptom complaints, should not only be tested for thyroid hormone levels and thyroid antibodies but should also have a complete blood count (CBC) and glucose levels (A1C) tests, to check for diabetes and other blood disorders."

(End of my reply.)

CHAPTER NINE

At What Point Does Thyroid Autoimmunity Cause Hypothyroidism?

The e-mail response below, I made to a woman writing to me about being diagnosed with thyroid autoimmunity. In other words, she was found to have killer cells attacking her thyroid gland, also called "thyroid antibodies". I went into some detail about these antibodies that cause thyroid disease and in how they correlate with development of hypothyroidism.

E-Mail Response:

"As you said in your e-mail, the "1120" (highly elevated) lab result you quoted was the TPO antibody or "anti-thyroidperoxidase", which is positive more commonly in people with autoimmune thyroid disease than the anti-thyroglobulin (TG) one is, when thyroid disease is caused by the immune system (thyroid autoimmunity). The immune system sends out these auto-antibodies to attack the thyroid gland because it has for some reason recognized it as an enemy in the body, as it normally would with germs, bacteria, fungus or allergens.

In some patients both antibodies can be highly positive but even if only the TPO is positive, this indicates autoimmune thyroid disease. Thyroid autoimmunity as it is also called is the most common cause of hypothyroidism in the US and other industrialized nations. The specific name of the autoimmune condition that causes hypothyroidism, due to the antibodies attacking the thyroid gland, is called "Hashimoto's thyroiditis".

I don't have your full story but if you are already being treated, you are just finding out the cause (autoimmune) of your hypothyroidism or at least the cause of your hypothyroid type symptoms. If you're not yet being treated, you likely will be soon but Doctors vary in what they consider the stage at which to treat a patient with thyroid autoimmunity, which is also showing signs of progressing into a hypothyroid state. Some factors involved in treatment decisions include the degree of symptoms being experienced and whether or not a goiter (thyroid enlargement) is present.

The "TSH" (Thyroid Stimulating Hormone), the pituitary hormone that monitors & stimulates thyroid hormone production will usually become abnormal first (it elevates with hypothyroidism) and afterward the thyroid hormones "T-3 and/or T-4" will begin to fall below the normal range as well. The TSH does the opposite and begins to elevate when a person's thyroid begins to fail. It is the hormone that stimulates the thyroid, so when it rises, that means it is having, to send an abnormally elevated amount to keep the thyroid working at proper level."

(End of my reply.)

CHAPTER TEN

Medical Research Agrees: Thyroid Autoimmunity Contributes to Symptoms

In this chapter, I will be commenting on a recently published medical research article about autoimmune thyroid disease. I would first like to make comments in regard to symptoms some patients with autoimmune hypothyroidism caused by Hashimoto's thyroiditis, experience that many medical Doctors will tell them, is not thyroid disease related.

Autoimmune hypothyroid patients will report to their Doctors, that they suffer systemic (system-wide or body-wide) joint and muscle aches. Patients will report experiencing neurological symptoms (nervous system) and sicca symptoms (areas of bodily dryness). These types of symptoms will be experienced by these patients even with their hypothyroidism being treated by hormone replacement therapy, to correct the low thyroid hormone levels. Their doctors will many times respond to their symptom complaints, by telling their patients that these type symptoms are not thyroid disease related but are rather emotionally based or imagined.

When further testing is then done and no further causes for their symptoms can be found, doctors will sometimes resort to the psychosomatic or emotional diagnosis. There is however more medical research being published, that clearly states that the autoimmune disease itself that causes hypothyroidism, is an additional cause of symptoms, apart from abnormal hormone levels.

In other words, the thyroid autoimmunity or disease process itself contributes to symptoms and may continue to do so, even after the low thyroid hormone levels from hypothyroidism, is corrected.

With my continual searching on the internet for new information about autoimmune thyroid disease, I occasionally run across medical research articles that stand out on particular subjects. In the case of the one I wish to comment on in this chapter, several technology publishing groups, have published conclusions by a medical research body; "Department of Pathophysiology, Medical School, National University of Athens, Greece", that looks at the subject of the "systemic manifestations" of autoimmune thyroid disease. It makes some statements that are in my opinion, very important for those in the medical community to make note of.

The research article is titled "Systemic Autoimmune Manifestations: When Should Underlying Thyroid Autoimmunity be Considered?" Within the abstract of this article that is indexed on search engines for public view, it states that this research group's clinical and laboratory data suggests that "thyroid autoimmunity" could be involved in the symptomology of these patients with systemic/rheumatic symptom manifestations.

The abstract also states that symptoms in these categories, such as musculoskeletal complaints and neurological manifestations, are not uncommon in patients with autoimmune thyroid disease, which affects 10% of the population.

39

In my opinion, this abstract/article which is published on the IngentaConnect.com website makes some extremely important observations and statements in regard to the role of thyroid autoimmunity in causing the symptoms of autoimmune thyroid disease.

With so much medical research and patient testimonials offered on the subject of the role of thyroid antibodies in both the thyroid disease process and its symptoms, doctors and patients alike should become better informed on this subject, as it relates to the effectiveness of hypothyroid treatment success.

(End - Section One)

SECTION TWO:

Cancer: A Great Concern for Thyroid Patients

Malignancies Affecting the Metabolic Butterfly

TABLE OF CONTENTS:

INTRODUCTION:

According to some medical information sources, thyroid disease is the most common of the endocrine diseases, including diabetes.

This is what the American Association of Clinical Endocrinologists (AACE) has to say about it:

"Thyroid disease is more common than diabetes or heart disease. Thyroid disease is a fact of life for as many as 27 million Americans – and more than half of those people remain undiagnosed."
(From Their "Empower" Website)
Source Link: http://www.empoweryourhealth.org/thyroid-conditions)

Many thyroid disease patients become aware of the fact that they are at an increased risk for developing thyroid malignancy but they are unsure how much that risk increases following diagnosis of their thyroid condition. Within the chapters of this book that follow, I offer information regarding these increased risk factors, backed by reputable medical information sources. Also included is information regarding thyroid cancer prevention, detection and treatments.

I believe this information may offer some comfort to thyroid disease patients but it will also help them to know what to look for regarding signs and symptoms of these higher-risk diseases and possibly to know what blood tests or other medical evaluations they may wish to request from their doctors should they suspect the possible onset of a malignant thyroid disease.

43

I am including quotes from medical research studies found on the U.S. National Institutes of Health website (reprints allowed for educational purposes).

Being aware of the medical possibilities and how they may manifest, through self-education, is part of what we in Thyroid Patient Advocacy refer-to as being "a proactive thyroid patient" and by doing so, one can help to secure a better quality of life for the sake of their selves and their families.

-Jim Lowrance

CHAPTER ONE

Can My Thyroid Disease Lead to Cancer in the Gland?

Most people who develop either hypothyroidism (underactive gland) or hyperthyroidism (overactive gland), do so as a result of "thyroid autoimmunity". This is the term that refers to the process in which auto-antibodies (destructive cells), attack the thyroid gland, rendering it incapable of producing proper amounts of thyroid hormone, to regulate metabolism within the cells of the body (the rate at which the body processes fuels coming into it for energy). Some research studies have shown an increased risk by people who have Grave's disease, for developing thyroid cancer of which the most common types are "follicular" and "papillary" malignancies ("medullary" and "anaplastic" are the less common types).

Following is a research study excerpt, published by the U.S. National Institutes of Health (PubMed), in regard to this risk:

"The relationship between Graves' disease or its therapy and carcinoma of the thyroid remains uncertain. We studied 20 patients found to have thyroid cancer in glands previously treated for Graves' disease between 1961 and 1986 at the University of Chicago Medical Center. Sixteen (80%) occurred in women and four (20%) occurred in men. The mean age at operation was 37 years (range, 19 to 69 years) and did not differ by sex. Fifteen of the 20 cancers (75%) were papillary while five (25%) were follicular. ---

Six individuals (30%) had a history of external radiation to the head and neck as an infant, child, or young adult. Two others had received radioiodine (RAI) therapy for Graves' disease 1 and 19 years earlier.

Patients were divided into three groups: group I: four patients (20%) had a neck mass 4, 14, 20, and 41 years after having had a subtotal thyroidectomy (STT) for Graves' disease; three of four had a history of external irradiation therapy. These tumors behaved aggressively, resulting in the death of two of the four patients. group II: 11 patients (55%) had diffusely enlarge toxic goiters without a nodule. A carcinoma was diagnosed intraoperatively on frozen section in only two of these patients. The others received STT. After recognition on permanent section, those carcinomas that were 4 mm or greater in diameter received postoperative RAI.

One recurrence occurred and was treated successfully with further RAI. group III: Five patients (25%) had Graves' disease and a palpable thyroid nodule. None of them had had a prior thyroidectomy for Graves' disease, as in group 1. Thyroid carcinoma was diagnosed in all patients preoperatively or intraoperatively, and a total thyroidectomy was performed. Each patient is alive and well with a mean follow-up of 5 years.

Between 1971 and 1981, 194 patients had surgery for Graves' disease, and 10 (5.2%) were found to have an associated carcinoma; six patients (3.1% of the total) did not have a nodule or any other suspicion of malignancy before surgery. ---

During the same time, 303 patients received RAI therapy for Graves' disease and one (0.3%) has subsequently developed thyroid carcinoma. Thyroid cancer associated with Graves' disease is found more commonly in surgically treated patients than in patients after RAI therapy.

The greatest risk factor in our patients was previous external radiation to the head and neck. Such individuals should be treated with total thyroid ablation rather than the usual STT, since they are at risk of developing aggressive thyroid cancers if thyroid remnants are left."

Source Link: http://www.ncbi.nlm.nih.gov/pubmed/3787468 ("Graves' disease and thyroid cancer.")

This particular study states that the risk for cancer in Graves' patients was more highly increased in those who underwent surgical subtotal thyroidectomies (SST -- partial removal of their glands), as opposed to those who had their thyroid glands ablated (destruction of it through radioactive iodine administration).

The research also points-out that the history of a significant percent of patient-participants in the study who developed thyroid cancer associated with their Graves' disease, had a history of external head and neck radiation as infants, during their childhoods, or during young adulthood (possibly referring mainly to frequent xrays).

Other Studies have shown an increased risk for ovarian cancer in women with Graves' disease as well.

47

A similar study published on the U.S. NIH, PubMed website, states that people with Hashimoto's disease (autoimmune thyroiditis that leads to hypothyroidism), are also at increased risk for developing thyroid cancer of the "papillary type" and that this risk is significantly higher in women than in men with the disease.
Following is a quote from that study:

*"**BACKGROUND:***

Hashimoto's thyroiditis (HT) is the most common cause of hypothyroidism and is characterized by gradual autoimmune mediated thyroid failure with occasional goiter development. HT is seven times more likely to occur in women than in men. Papillary thyroid cancer (PTC), the most prevalent form of cancer in the thyroid, is 2.5 times more likely to develop in women than men. Given the relatively high prevalence of these diseases and the increased occurrence in women, we analyzed data from our institution to determine if there is a correlation between Hashimoto's thyroiditis and PTC in women.

METHODS:

From May 1994 to January 2007, 1198 patients underwent thyroid surgery at our institution. Of these, 217 patients were diagnosed with HT (196 women, 21 men). The data from these patients were statistically analyzed using SPSS.

RESULTS:

PTC occurred in 63 of 217 (29%) HT patients and 230 of 981 (23%) patients without HT (P = 0.051). ---

Of these groups, 41 (65%) and 158 (69%) patients, respectively, had tumor sizes >/=1.0 cm; 56/196 women (29%) with HT had coexistent PTC compared with 160/730 women (22%) without HT (P = 0.03). Among women with any type of thyroid malignancy, 56/59 cases (95%) with HT had PTC compared with 159/196 cases (81%) in women without HT (P = 0.006). Additionally, female HT patients with goiters had a significantly lower rate of PTC (9% versus 36%, P < 0.001) compared with women without goiters. These differences were not observed in men with HT.

CONCLUSIONS:

These data demonstrate that HT is associated with an increased risk of developing PTC. Female patients with HT undergoing thyroidectomy are 30% more likely to have PTC. Thus, more aggressive surveillance for PTC may be indicated in patients with HT, especially in women."

Source Link:
http://www.ncbi.nlm.nih.gov/pubmed/17996901
("Hashimoto's thyroiditis a risk factor for papillary thyroid cancer?")

CHAPTER TWO

Can Diet Nutritional Supplementation and Exercise Really Protect Against Thyroid Cancer Risks?

Certainly, a recommendation that is always given to thyroid patients by their doctors is to live the healthiest lives possible, to include proper diet and exercise. The exercise aspect is somewhat obvious and self-explanatory and would include the warning that one should exercise only to tolerance-level and to not overdo when undertaking a regimen, whether of the aerobic or strength and endurance types.

Research studies have shown that exercise does indeed lower the risk for cancer development of all types, as does getting proper rest and sleep and so this is one of those obvious things that is available to practically everyone who is healthy enough to exercise regularly.

Research regarding exercise and breast cancer risk reduction (would also obviously apply to other types largely affecting women, including thyroid cancers):

"BACKGROUND:

Epidemiologic evidence strongly suggests that cumulative exposure to ovarian hormones is a determinant of breast cancer risk. Because physical activity can modify menstrual cycle patterns and alter the production of ovarian hormones, it may reduce breast cancer risk; yet few epidemiologic studies have assessed this relationship.

50

PURPOSE:

The major objective of this study was to determine whether young women (aged 40 and younger) who regularly participated in physical exercise activities during their reproductive years had a reduced risk of breast cancer.

METHODS:

Using a case-control design, we conducted personal interviews of a total of 545 women (aged 40 and younger at diagnosis) who had been newly diagnosed with in situ or invasive breast cancer between July 1, 1983, and January 1, 1989, and a total of 545 control subjects. Case patients and control subjects were individually matched on date of birth (within 36 months), race (white), parity (nulliparous versusparous), and neighborhood of residence. Lifetime histories of participation in physical exercise activities on a regular basis were obtained during the personal interview.

RESULTS:

After adjustment for potential confounding factors, we found that the average number of hours spent in physical exercise activities per week from menarche to 1 year prior to the case patient's diagnosis was a significant predictor of reduced breast cancer risk (two-sided P for trend < . 0001). The odds ratio (OR) of breast cancer among women who, on average, spent 3.8 or more hours per week participating in physical exercise activities was 0.42 (95% confidence limits [CLs] = 0.27, 0.64) relative to inactive women. ---

The effect was stronger among women who had had a full-term pregnancy. Comparing most active (> or = 3.8 hours/wk of exercise) women to inactive women, the ORs were 0.28 (95% CL = 0.16, 0.50) for parous and 0.73 (95% CL = 0.38, 1.41) for nulliparous women.

CONCLUSIONS:

Most previously identified risk factors for breast cancer are reproductive and menstrual events that cannot be readily altered. The protective effect of exercise on breast cancer risk in the women whom we studied suggests that physical activity offers one modifiable lifestyle characteristic that may substantially reduce a woman's lifetime risk of breast cancer.

IMPLICATIONS:

Whether the protective effects of exercise on breast cancer risk are due to alterations in ovarian function and whether they extend into women's menopausal years need to be established. Our results suggest that implementation of regular physical exercise programs as a critical component of a healthy lifestyle should be a high priority for adolescent and adult women."

Source Link: http://www.ncbi.nlm.nih.gov/pubmed/8072034 ("Physical exercise and reduced risk of breast cancer in young women.")

The diet aspect of reducing cancer risk would of course include the recommendation to avoid junk foods (simple carbohydrates -- foods high in saturated fats and high levels of manufactured sugars).

The goal is to eat healthy, complex carbohydrates (fruits, vegetables, nuts and grains) however, thyroid patients should avoid certain types of foods that in the long run, can help the thyroid gland to not suffer as severely from autoimmunity that contributes to worsening thyroiditis and hypothyroidism. This would include the avoidance of "goitrogen foods" of which "soy" is a major one and that can be a by-product found in many food-products but is often not recognized unless ingredients are carefully read on food product labels (i.e. soybeans, tofu, soybean oil, soy flour, soy lecithin).

Other goitrogen foods include the following:

• cassava
• Pine nuts
• Peanuts
• Millet
• Strawberries
• Pears
• Peaches
• Spinach
• Bamboo shoots
• Sweet Potatoes
• Bok choy
• Broccoli
• Broccolini (Asparations)
• Brussels sprouts
• Cabbage
• Canola
• Cauliflower
• Chinese cabbage
• Choy sum
• Collard greens ---

- Horseradish
- Kai-lan (Chinese broccoli)
- Kale
- Kohlrabi
- Mizuna
- Mustard greens
- Radishes
- Rapeseed (yu choy)
- Rapini
- Rutabagas
- Tatsoi
- Turnips

Some medical sources state that the goitrogen effect of these foods, can be reduced considerably when they are cooked properly (those that require cooking) and when those who have thyroid disease, consume them in moderation (especially those foods that don't require being cooked).

Healthy versus Unhealthy Fats

An additional note in regard to "saturated fats" as mentioned previously -- these are the unhealthy dietary types, while there are healthy dietary fats called "monounsaturated and polyunsaturated" and these actually help to lower any bad fat levels in the body that can lead to high cholesterol. One method for making sure that one is taking ample amounts of healthy fat in the diet is by supplementing with "omega-3 fats" (fish oil) found in over-the-counter caplets available in the natural supplements departments of department stores and health shops.

This can help to raise the "HDL" cholesterol level (the healthy type), which can decrease any harmful effects from elevated "LDL" cholesterol levels (the unhealthy type).

Following is a research study quote, in regard to healthy cholesterol levels, decreasing prostate cancer risks in males and how statin medications may help in this area, when need (logically also true of other types of cancers):

"BACKGROUND:

Studies suggest a decreased risk of high-grade prostate cancer in men with lower circulating total cholesterol and that statins may protect against aggressive disease. Confirmation in additional populations and examination of associations for lipoprotein subfractions are needed.

METHODS:

We examined prostate cancer risk and serum total and HDL cholesterol in the ATBC Study cohort (n = 29,093). Cox proportional hazards models were used to estimate the relative risk of total (n = 2,041), non-aggressive (n = 829), aggressive (n = 461), advanced (n = 412), and high-grade (n = 231) prostate cancer by categories of total and HDL cholesterol.

RESULTS:

After excluding the first 10 years of follow-up, men with higher serum total cholesterol were at increased risk of overall ($\geq$240 vs. <200 mg/dl: HR = 1.22, 95% CI 1.03-1.44, p-trend = 0.01) and advanced ($\geq$240 vs. <200 mg/dl: HR = 1.85, 95% CI 1.13-3.03, p-trend = 0.05) prostate cancer. ---

Higher HDL cholesterol was suggestively associated with a decreased risk of prostate cancer regardless of stage or grade.

CONCLUSIONS:

In this population of smokers, high serum total cholesterol was associated with higher risk of advanced prostate cancer, and high HDL cholesterol suggestively reduced the risk of prostate cancer overall.These results support previous studies and, indirectly, support the hypothesis that statins may reduce the risk of advanced prostate cancer by lowering cholesterol."

Source Link:
http://www.ncbi.nlm.nih.gov/pubmed/21915616 ("Serum total and HDL cholesterol and risk of prostate cancer.")

Other Healthy Supplements that Decrease Thyroid Cancer Risk

According to a great deal of medical research that is available, nutritional supplements can indeed offset the risk for cancer development of all types. Some studies have shown that essential vitamins becoming deficient can significantly increase the chances for cancer developing. This includes a vitamin that has become deficient in the American public as well as in third world countries of the world and this would be the all-important "vitamin D".

Following is one research study from Pubmed/U.S. NIH, to this effect:

"*PURPOSE:*

Higher serum levels of the main circulating form of vitamin D, 25-hydroxyvitamin D (25(OH)D), are associated with substantially lower incidence rates of colon, breast, ovarian, renal, pancreatic, aggressive prostate and other cancers.

METHODS:

Epidemiological findings combined with newly discovered mechanisms suggest a new model of cancer etiology that accounts for these actions of 25(OH)D and calcium. Its seven phases are disjunction, initiation, natural selection, overgrowth, metastasis, involution, and transition (abbreviated DINOMIT). Vitamin D metabolites prevent disjunction of cells and are beneficial in other phases.

RESULTS/CONCLUSIONS:

It is projected that raising the minimum year-around serum 25(OH)D level to 40 to 60 ng/mL (100-150 nmol/L) would prevent approximately 58,000 new cases of breast cancer and 49,000 new cases of colorectal cancer each year, and three fourths of deaths from these diseases in the United States and Canada, based on observational studies combined with a randomized trial. Such intakes also are expected to reduce case-fatality rates of patients who have breast, colorectal, or prostate cancer by half. There are no unreasonable risks from intake of 2000 IU per day of vitamin D(3), or from a population serum 25(OH)D level of 40 to 60 ng/mL. The time has arrived for nationally coordinated action to substantially increase intake of vitamin D and calcium."

Source Link:
http://www.ncbi.nlm.nih.gov/pubmed/19523595 ("Vitamin D for cancer prevention: global perspective.")

Note that this research states that taking up to "2,000 IU of vitamin D per day", is not considered over-supplementation however, many doctors recommend approximately "1,000 IU per day", unless a severe deficiency is found and in these cases, mega-doses may be required for a period of time.

Getting Blood Tested for Nutritional Deficiencies

All thyroid patients should undergo testing of major vitamin levels (i.e. D, B12, E and B6) and other nutrients (i.e. minerals, protein and electrolyte levels) because deficiencies can be present, without necessarily causing any suggestive symptoms. If vitamin levels or other nutrients are found to be deficient, further testing should also be done, to find if there are malabsorption syndromes present as well. These are disorders, in which nutrients are hindered in the body and organs cannot utilize them properly, which can include the digestive tract and the liver. Diseases of these organs, resulting in nutritional malabsorption, can include Celiac disease (intolerance to gluten in the diet) and types of liver disease, such as viral and autoimmune hepatitis. If such diseases are found, supplementation with the needed nutrients that are deficient, in addition to treating the underlying disease process would become necessary. If deficiencies only are found, with no particular cause behind them (idiopathic), supplementing them to bring them back up to proper levels, can be highly beneficial, not only as a cancer preventative but for overall better health as well.

CHAPTER THREE

Supplementing with Selenium

One nutrient that has also been covered in medical research studies, regarding supplements that can decrease thyroid disease activity, is "selenium", which is both a mineral and an electrolyte that is essential in the body. According to these research studies, the mineral actually "modifies" levels of the antibodies that cause thyroid diseases as discussed earlier. The two major thyroid antibodies, also called "auto-antibodies", that attack key proteins within the gland, causing diseases such as Hashimoto's thyroiditis and Graves' disease, are the "anti-thyroidperoxidase" (immune cells that attack thethyroidperoxidase enzyme/protein – abbreviated "Anti-TPO") and the "anti-thyroglobulin" (immune cells that attack the thyroglobulin enzyme/protein – abbreviated anti-TG).

Selenium, supplemented as a daily regimen, is cited in these studies as having the ability to reduce the TPO antibodies, thereby reducing disease activity in the thyroid gland and the associated inflammation that is also involved. Additionally, other research studies state that it can also reduce the risk for cancers of the lung, colorectal, and prostate types.

Research citing selenium as a cancer risk reducer:

"Studies examining the relationship between dietary selenium intake and risk of various cancers have shown that low selenium intake is associated with higher cancer rates. ---

A recent well-controlled intervention trial studied whether selenium supplementation can prevent cancer in subjects who have a history of skin cancer and live in areas of the United States with low soil selenium levels. Selenium supplementation did not reduce skin cancer rates, but the incidence of total, lung, colorectal, and prostate cancers was significantly reduced by the intervention. Although these data need confirmation, they suggest that adequate selenium intake is essential for cancer prevention."

Source Link:
http://www.ncbi.nlm.nih.gov/pubmed/9279064 ("Dietary selenium repletion may reduce cancer incidence in people at high risk who live in areas with low soil selenium.")

Research citing selenium as a modifier of thyroid autoimmunity activity:

"In areas with severe selenium deficiency there is a higher incidence of thyroiditis due to a decreased activity of selenium-dependent glutathione peroxidase activity within thyroid cells. Selenium-dependent enzymes also have several modifying effects on the immune system. Therefore, even mild selenium deficiency may contribute to the development and maintenance of autoimmune thyroid diseases.

We performed a blinded, placebo-controlled, prospective study in female patients (n = 70; mean age, 47.5 +/- 0.7 yr) with autoimmune thyroiditis and thyroid peroxidase antibodies (TPOAb) and/or Tgantibodies (TgAb) above 350 IU/ml. The primary end point of the study was the change in TPOAb concentrations. ---

Secondary end points were changes in TgAb, TSH, and free thyroid hormone levels as well asultrasound pattern of the thyroid and quality of life estimation.

Patients were randomized into 2 age- and antibody (TPOAb)-matched groups; 36 patients received 200 microg (2.53 micromol) sodium selenite/d, orally, for 3 months, and 34 patients received placebo. All patients were substituted with L-T(4) to maintain TSH within the normal range. TPOAb, TgAb, TSH, and free thyroid hormones were determined by commercial assays. The echogenicity of the thyroid was monitored with high resolution ultrasound. The mean TPOAb concentration decreased significantly to 63.6% (P = 0.013) in the selenium group vs. 88% (P = 0.95) in the placebo group.

A subgroup analysis of those patients with TPOAb greater than 1200 IU/ml revealed a mean 40% reduction in the selenium-treated patients compared with a 10% increase in TPOAb in the placebo group.TgAb concentrations were lower in the placebo group at the beginning of the study and significantly further decreased (P = 0.018), but were unchanged in the selenium group.

Nine patients in the selenium-treated group had completely normalized antibody concentrations, in contrast to two patients in the placebo group (by chi(2) test, P = 0.01). Ultrasound of the thyroid showed normalized echogenicity in these patients. The mean TSH, free T(4), and free T(3) levels were unchanged in both groups. We conclude that selenium substitution may improve the inflammatory activity in patients with autoimmune thyroiditis, especially in those with high activity. ---

Whether this effect is specific for autoimmune thyroiditis or may also be effective in other endocrine autoimmune diseases has yet to be investigated."

Source Link:
http://www.ncbi.nlm.nih.gov/pubmed/11932302 (Selenium supplementation in patients with autoimmune thyroiditis decreases thyroid peroxidase antibodies concentrations.")

The conclusions that can be derived from the combination of these two previously quoted medical studies, is that both thyroid autoimmunity and cancers that can potentially affect the thyroid gland, can both be modified and/or reduced in risk for development, through selenium supplementation. It is always recommended however, that dosing directions are followed according to a manufacturers label and that the supplement is reported to one's doctor, to make sure it cannot potentially contraindicate (interfere) with other medications or supplements that are already being taken.

CHAPTER FOUR

Monitoring for Thyroid Cancer Symptoms

The symptoms of thyroid cancer can be non-specific and often, there are no symptoms to indicate that the disease is present. When symptoms do occur, they usually involve discomfort of various types, in the throat.

A person with thyroid malignancy developing may find that they are having throat pain that can be felt when turning their head or stretching their neck with body position changes and/or they may feel soreness inside their throat that manifests like a typical sore throat that occurs with colds, viral illnesses or allergies. The difference being that a sore throat that occurs with thyroid cancer does not usually get better but will worsen over time.

Thyroid cancer can also cause voice changes such as hoarseness or a deeper tone to one's voice due to any constriction present from swelling or tumors requiring more effort to project words. When thyroid tumors, also called "nodules" increase in size with malignancy, they can cause a person to experience difficulty swallowing or even breathing difficulties if they become large enough.

Other than these aforementioned symptoms affecting the throat, other indirect symptoms of thyroid malignancy can occur rarely, including fever or anemia (if blood loss is involved) but in many cases, the disease develops with no noticeable symptoms being present.

Self Palpating (Examining) the Thyroid Gland

With the fact of thyroid cancer not causing symptoms in many cases, thyroid disease patients can perform home self-exams, of their glands and report any noticeable changes in size or texture that may occur within it, to their doctors. While a person can sometimes detect a goiter and/or thyroid nodules by self examination, a definitive diagnoses must be given by a qualified physician.

Abnormalities in size and/or texture of the thyroid gland can occur with both hypothyroid and hyperthyroid conditions but are more common in autoimmune thyroid diseases. As previously stated, this can also be the case with thyroid malignancy as well. If a person feels he may be experiencing thyroid-related symptoms or has detected an abnormal feeling in their thyroid gland, a preliminary self-examination can be done while an appointment with a qualified physician has been scheduled.
A patient can then report any findings that indicate problems in the gland to his medical doctor. The eMedicine/WebMD website states in their article titled "Goiter Nontoxic: Follow-Up", under the Patient Education sub-heading that "Thyroid self-examination may be taught to patients, allowing them to monitor their own body for early changes in gland size."

Palpating the Thyroid Gland

A person can feel his own throat, using the fingertips (palpation), in the area of the thyroid gland, to detect swelling or lumps. The thyroid is located in the center of the throat, directly beneath the Adams apple.

In males it is more prominent but can usually be located easily in females as well. Once finding the Adams apple, the isthmus (middle portion) of the thyroid is only about an inch or, slightly lower below it and will be slightly raised. If the isthmus protrudes significantly, or feels very firm to the touch, this can indicate a goiter or thyroid nodule being present in that portion of the gland.

Shape of the Gland

There are also two lobes of the thyroid gland, one of each side of it, that extend about an inch toward the inside of the throat and that extend upward toward the Adams apple, about even with it. The gland is typically small and forms a butterfly shape. The lobes actually attach to the Adams apple and throat with connecting cartilage and tissue but when they are normal size, are usually not easily felt unless pressed-on firmly with the fingertips. If they are easily detectable without firmly pressing down on them or are visible without the need to palpate them, this can indicate a goiter or nodules in the lobe-areas as well.

The Swallow Test

While palpation is being done to detect swelling (enlargement) in the gland, any lumps or protrusions that might indicate a thyroid nodule (tumor-like growth) or several of them should also be checked for. These can also be spotted by tilting the head back, while looking in a mirror and taking sips of water, watching for any signs of enlargement or lumps as the gland moves up and down in the throat. Some people with enlarged glands are found to have both goiter and nodules, which is referred to as a "nodular goiter" or a "multi-nodular goiter".

Difficulty Swallowing

If a person feels a lump on the inside of his throat when swallowing, this can indicate a thyroid nodule that is growing toward the inside and that cannot be felt from the outside of the throat. If there is a general feeling of difficulty swallowing or breathing due to the throat being constricted, this may also indicate a goiter in which the enlargement is swelling toward the inside of the throat. This type problem is not always indicative of thyroid problems but can be related to esophagus problems as well.

If any of these self-examination methods are found to indicate a problem in the gland, it should be reported to a medical doctor as soon as possible for further evaluation.

Thyroid Cancer Diagnostic Tests

While blood abnormalities would actually be considered a "sign" rather than a "symptom" of thyroid cancer, there are several of these that can be ordered for someone suspected of having possibly malignancy in their thyroid gland. These tests would include a "Complete Blood Count", which evaluates the red and white blood cells, to see if there is a decrease or change in the size of them. With cancer of any kind the total white blood cell count (leukocytes) will often increase, which is a condition known as "leukocytosis" or with certain types of cancer, it may actually decrease (i.e. with lymphoma and leukemia), which is referred to as "leukopenia". Adversely the total red blood cells (erythrocytes) may decrease if blood loss has begun to occur with cancers of any kind (anemia).

Inflammatory markers in the blood can increase when cancer is present as well but may also do-so simply due to highly active thyroid autoimmunity (i.e. C-Reactive Protein and the Erythrocyte Sedimentation Rate levels).

Two blood tests that are more specific to thyroid cancer diagnosis are the "calcitonin" and "thyroglobulin" levels. These substances will become elevated in the blood, in some cases of thyroid cancer types. They are also used for follow-up tests after treatment for thyroid malignancy has been administered to monitor progress of the treatment.

In some cases, a thyroid biopsy will be performed to detect or to rule out cancer being present within the gland. Some patients are given a "fine needle aspiration" biopsy, which is usually an out-patient test in which a hypodermic needle is inserted into the gland, to extract small amounts of tissue for analysis. Other patients may be referred for a surgical biopsy in which a larger area of tissue is removed while they are under full anesthesia. Yet other patients may be sent for imaging tests of their thyroid glands, such as "thyroid ultrasound" and "MRI" (magnetic resonance imaging) or a "CT Scan" (multiple-angle radiograph images).

CHAPTER FIVE

Thyroid Cancer Treatments

When a patient is confirmed as having thyroid cancer, via the medical tests that diagnose it, the treating doctor will refer the patient to a surgeon, who will determine how the cancer will need to be removed. If the cancer affects only one of the two lobes of the thyroid, the surgeon may wish to perform what is called a "lobectomy", (partial thyroidectomy) meaning there will be removal of only one side of the gland.

If the surgeon feels removal of only one lobe, still places the patient at risk for the cancer returning, he may instead decide to remove the entire gland, which is referred to as a "total thyroidectomy". The type surgery is also determined by considering the type of thyroid cancer that is involved. Some types of cancer are more aggressive than others and with these the surgeon will always recommend total thyroid removal. Surgeons also must determine at what stage the cancer is in, meaning how far it has progressed.

In order to decrease the risk of the cancer returning, the surgeon may also want to remove the lymph nodes in the neck, that are located near the thyroid gland. The lymph nodes may also be sent off for laboratory analysis to determine if they already contained cancer, which might then lead the surgeon to recommend further treatment(s).

Post Operative Thyroid Cancer Treatments

Additional treatment after any type of thyroidectomy might also include Radio Active Iodine Therapy (RAI) or Chemotherapy.

This is to destroy any remaining thyroid tissue that is capable of absorbing iodine in the body or any remaining cancer cells. Any remaining thyroid tissue that is capable of taking up iodine, which is what the thyroid mainly consists of, also has the ability to re-develop cancer cells and is the reason RAI is sometimes used following a Total Thyroidectomy. Chemotherapy is directed at any remaining cancer cells that might remain in the body after a Total Thyroidectomy.

Regardless of the type of thyroid surgery that is performed, thyroid hormone replacement therapy is always used following thyroid cancer surgeries.

The goal of the hormone therapy is to suppress the patient's TSH level, which decreases when thyroid hormone is increased via a hormone dose. This also helps prevent recurrence of cancer but also replaces any hormone the thyroid gland is not capable of producing following surgery (hypothyroidism).

If a patient is given RAI after surgery, they may not be replaced with thyroid hormone for a month or two following the treatment. Most patients will need thyroid hormone replacement therapy following any type of thyroidectomy, as lifelong treatment.

The treating Doctor will prescribe a starting dose of thyroid hormone for the patient and will order follow-up blood re-testing to adjust the dose to the correct level over time, which is called "titrating" the dose. Each new dose level takes about eight weeks to fully adjust in the body.

Following are helpful suggestions for patients who are placed on thyroid hormone therapy following thyroid cancer treatment:

• Take your thyroid hormone medication on an empty stomach, with plenty of water.
• Take your thyroid hormone medication at the same time each day.
• If you take vitamins or supplements containing iron or calcium, be sure to take them six hours apart from your thyroid medication dose.
• When you have blood retests of your thyroid hormone levels, take your medication at the same time, to correlate with each blood draw.
• Never adjust your own thyroid medication dose.

Thyroid cancers have a very high treatment success rate but that success rate is even higher when thyroid cancers are diagnosed and treated as early as possible.

It is very important to see your doctor if you discover any nodules (tumor-like growths) on your thyroid gland or if you have difficulty swallowing, a chronic sore throat or feel, that you might have a growth on the inside of your throat.

(END - Section two)

SECTION THREE

Common Thyroid Disease Complications

Secondary Problems Needing Special Attention

INTRODUCTION:

There are basically two categories of thyroid dysfunction, the one being an under-active thyroid gland or "hypothyroidism" and the other being an overactive thyroid gland or "hyperthyroidism". Both conditions of thyroid hormone imbalance can develop due to a number of different causes and both have treatments that can return the abnormally high or abnormally low levels of thyroid hormones, back-to the normal values range (optimally when possible). The goal of these treatments is to restore a patient's bodily metabolism, so that it functions at the best possible level.

While a patient may see their thyroid dysfunction resolved over time, they may potentially experience secondary complications of their thyroid diseases that will require special attention and/or additional treatments. In this book, I will be addressing a number of these type issues, many being common thyroid disease complications with others being less common or rare. It is important that thyroid patients be made aware of both the common and rare types of complications because some of these have better treatment outcomes, the earlier they can be diagnosed and treated.

72

TABLE OF CONTENTS

CHAPTER ONE

Hair Loss

A symptom that is listed for both hypothyroid and hyperthyroid conditions is "hair loss". Some patients, especially those with hyperthyroidism, may see rapid hair loss with their thyroid disorder. Other patients only see mild to moderate hair loss, such as finding more hair in the sink after washing it. Hypothyroid patients will find that their hair becomes dry and brittle and will also break off rather than just falling out. Some thyroid patients being treated for hypothyroidism will report that they experience hair loss, more so with a particular type of thyroid hormone replacement medication. The hair loss they experienced prior to starting hormone therapy was mild to moderate or in some cases almost unnoticeable but once starting thyroid medication, they see a rapid increase in hair loss. I have seen this attested to, more often in patients taking synthetic forms of thyroid hormone medications, while other patients are not affected in regard to hair loss by synthetic or the natural types (animal derived) of thyroid hormone medications.

In my case, as a hypothyroid patient, I experienced mild hair loss when I began to experience symptoms of hypothyroidism from Hashimoto's thyroiditis (autoimmune disease - the most common cause in industrialized countries). I would find a half dozen or so hairs in my sink after hair washing and possibly a few hairs on my pillow upon waking but I did not see moderate or severe hair loss. At one point during my thyroid hormone therapy, I was switched from Armour brand, natural thyroid medication to Thyrolar, a synthetic combination T-4/T-3 medication.

After about two weeks on Thyrolar, my hair began to fall out in moderate amounts. I actually was only switched from Armour, to see if mild intermittent hives I was experiencing were due to it but after over a month on Thyrolar, the mild hives continued and so the hives were attributed to my thyroid autoimmunity and not caused by the type thyroid medication I was taking. With this being the case I asked to be switched back to Armour and the hair loss stopped.

Patients are individuals and none of the scenarios I described are true of everyone. It is also true that most patients taking a type of thyroid medication that does cause them hair loss will see this side effect resolve given additional adjustment time on their thyroid hormone therapy. One importance in the hair loss symptom in people, who are not on thyroid hormone therapy, is recognizing the fact that it can be an indication of thyroid hormone imbalance, especially in people who are experiencing other symptoms that may indicate a change in their thyroid function.

CHAPTER TWO

Diminished Libido

There are many concerning symptoms that can occur with thyroid disease but one of the more concerning ones is loss of libido or a decreased sex drive. One reason this particular symptom can be so concerning is because of the possible strain it can place on the marriage of a thyroid patient (whether real or perceived). I know this concern to be a very real one because I have corresponded with both male and female patients with this problem and concern on thyroid forums, repeatedly over the years since year-2003. It is such a great concern to some of them, that it causes them increased depression symptoms as well.

Patients with more of a problem with loss of libido are those with hypothyroidism. Those with hyperthyroidism can also experience this symptom but they can also experience episodes of increased sex drive, due to the sped up metabolism hyperthyroidism can cause. With hypothyroidism, the metabolism is slowed down, which means the reproductive organs are slowed down as well. The adrenal glands that produce precursor hormones that convert into the sex hormones are also slowed down and both men and women can see decreased testosterone and estrogen levels. Both males and females have both of these sex hormones in their bodies but in different balance for each.

The good news is that when thyroid hormone imbalances of either type are corrected, the result is a normalizing of all bodily functions, including the sex drive.

Many thyroid patients report that they regain a certain degree of their libido back although many, report that it is not restored to 100%, as it was before thyroid disease. To regain a significant percentage however is far better than to remain in an almost void state of libido that some patients report.

There are also prescription drugs that can help men in this area and the reason this is slightly more of a concern for men, is due to the fact that they rely upon a bodily function that if not operating properly, prevents intimacy with their partner from taking place. This fact is also the reason lack of libido can seriously affect some men psychologically because they feel lack of ability to perform sexually, brings into question, their masculinity and ability to satisfy their partner. In some cases, this can then lead them to worry about their marriage in general.

Certainly this is also a concern to women who also have problems with being responsive to their husbands, due to decreased libido. In addition to drugs that can help, there are also hormone therapies that can be administered by a treating Doctor, if the sex hormones are found to be low and in need of additional hormone therapies to correct them.

Thyroid hormone therapy must sometimes be given several months time to help in areas such as libido because it can take this much time to see all bodily organs regain a significant degree of their pre-disease functions. If libido is not adequately restored with thyroid hormone replacement, patients should remember that their Doctors may be able to suggest additional drug or hormone therapies as described above, that can help in this area.

CHAPTER THREE

Thyroid Autoimmunity and Hives-Rash (Uticaria)

In recent years, medical research has found a strong connection between thyroid autoimmunity and hives or what is medically known as "chronic uticaria". Some of the studies specifically state that "Hashimoto's thyroiditis" can be a cause of recurrent hives. Yet even more medical research studies have shown that children with chronic hives or uticaria should be screened for autoimmune thyroid disease by blood testing their thyroid hormone levels and also testing them for "thyroid antibodies".

The two types of thyroid antibodies (also called auto-antibodies), that are most common in causing autoimmune thyroid disease are the "anti-thyroidperoxidase" antibodies (TPO) and the "anti-thyroglobulin" antibodies (TG). If either or both of these are found to be positive in patients with chronic hives, this could be an explanation for their cause.

When I was diagnosed with hypothyroidism, in early 2003, one of the symptoms I experienced that told me something unusual was occurring in my body, was a severe case of hives I experienced, just before worsening symptoms of hypothyroidism, also began to occur.

I had never experienced uticaria previous to this from either allergies or stress and I felt they were a strong indication that something serious was going on with my immune system.

It was in fact thyroid auto-immunity that was flaring up in my system and the hives were a result of this chronic immune response that was destroying my thyroid gland and causing me to also experience progressive hypothyroidism (under-active thyroid).

The doctor I visited when the hives were flaring up, felt that I was experiencing a food allergy but this had never happened before and I instead thought it was an allergy to a plant of some type because I had been doing a lot of landscape work at that time, while managing some property. The job I had at the time was also very stressful and so I also considered the severe stress as a possibility. The fact is however that I was experiencing the onset of hypothyroidism, from Hashimoto's thyroiditis.

I feel the disease hit a level of severity, with stress as a possible contributing factor that caused my body to release histamine (fluid produced by the immune system, to fight allergens) which surfaced on my skin, as a severe case of uticaria.

The PubMed medical research website, provided by the National Institutes of Health and the National Library of Medicine, published an article entitled; "Association between chronic urticaria and thyroid autoimmunity: a prospective study involving 99 patients."

The article states the following conclusion; *"This study shows a significant association between chronic urticaria and thyroid autoimmunity, and that tests to detect thyroid autoantibodies are relevant in patients with chronic urticaria, whereas extensive laboratory tests are not."*

When chronic hives (uticaria) is experienced and is an unusual occurrence not easily explained by an allergen or another obvious cause, a patient should see their doctor and request thyroid antibodies and thyroid function tests to be ordered. These tests can rule out thyroid autoimmunity or help confirm it as being the cause of this condition.

CHAPTER FOUR

Peripheral Neuropathy

Many thyroid patients complain of neurological type symptoms and many struggle with these despite the fact that they are well treated to correct their thyroid hormone imbalance. In addition to thyroid disorders, other endocrine diseases, such as diabetes can cause symptoms of neuropathy, as can neurological disorders that originate in the brain. "Peripheral Neuropathy" is a term meaning a patient suffers from nerve-related symptoms in their body. These can affect nerves that travel to other parts of the body, so that there is a systemic or referred type effect, meaning there are many areas of the body being affected.

The symptoms of neuropathies can include tingling and numbness sensations in the body but the extremities are more commonly affected (hands and feet). It can also include burning sensations, muscle weakness and stabbing type pains.

Muscle twitches and tremor in the muscles can also be a common symptom of peripheral neuropathy (fasciculations). This particular one affects many thyroid patients with Grave's Disease but can also manifest in those with Hashimoto's thyroiditis.

Some patients with neuropathy type symptoms will also complain of tinnitus, meaning they experience ringing, roaring or clicking sounds in their ears. Some may also experience a degree of hearing loss and dizziness caused by the imbalanced nerve signals reaching the inner ears.

In the year 2007, I had a Brain MRI performed, due to experiencing the symptoms I describe above. My test result came back negative for signs of neurological disease and this confirmed to me that my peripheral neuropathy was likely caused or at least aggravated by my autoimmune thyroid disease.

Some medical sources state that neurological symptoms are rare in thyroid disease patients with hypothyroidism however this is not what I've been hearing from 100s of patients over the years who attest to experiencing neuropathies, despite being well treated. My belief is that these symptoms may originate from thyroid auto-antibody levels and not from thyroid hormone imbalance alone.

There is a severe thyroid antibody condition called "Hashimoto's Encephalitis" (also referred-to as "Hashimoto's Encephalopathy") that causes severe neurological symptoms and is caused by thyroid antibodies (thyroid autoimmunity) however; it is a very rare disorder. It can present with epileptic seizures, amnesia, psychosis and even coma or death. I feel there are lesser degrees of thyroid antibody related peripheral neuropathy and that it is only common sense to recognize that they can cause neuropathies that are milder than those of Hashimoto's Encephalitis. More on this condition will be addressed in 'CHAPTER FIFTEEN'.

If you are a thyroid patient experiencing peripheral neuropathy symptoms, discuss with your doctor any testing you might need, to rule out causes other than your treated thyroid disease.

Online medical research links that mention Thyroid Disease as a cause of peripheral neuropathy includes the following:

http://www.ninds.nih.gov/disorders/peripheralneuropathy/detail_peripheralneuropathy.htm *(National Institute of Neurological Disorders and Stroke)*

http://www.emedicine.com/neuro/TOPIC214.HTM *(WebMD)*

http://www.pubmedcentral.nih.gov/articlerender.fcgi?artid=1031603 *(PubMed)*

http://www.neurology.org/cgi/content/abstract/67/5/786*(American Academy of Neurology)*

CHAPTER FIVE

Joint and Muscle Pain

Over the past few years, I have corresponded with many thyroid patients with Hashimoto's Disease, the autoimmune type hypothyroidism. Patients with the disease complain of many symptoms they experience with this disease that are caused by antibodies attacking the thyroid gland, causing it to hypo-function but one of the more common ones I hear repeated by patients, is mild to moderate "joint and muscle pain".

This particular symptom is also one of those that can seem to linger in some patients, months or even years after starting treatment for their hypothyroidism, with hormone replacement medication.

Strangely, some patients actually experience a worsening of their joint/muscle pain, once beginning thyroid medication and this was the experience I personally had, after beginning treatment with hormone replacement for Hashimoto's Hypothyroidism.

I cannot explain this particular phenomenon but know for a fact, patients do experience it, until their bodies adjust completely to their thyroid medication.

What aspect of this disease, results in the concerning symptoms that affect the patient's joints and muscles? There are many contributing factors however, I believe two of the main causes, are inflammation and decreased blood circulation, from slowed metabolism.

The inflammation aspect is from the autoimmune process that causes antibodies to attack the thyroid gland, resulting in high levels of inflammation. This inflammation first affects the area of the thyroid gland itself but it is my belief, that over time, continuing inflammation is going to eventually have a systemic affect and travel to other parts of the body.

I also believe it is no coincidence that autoimmune disease thyroid patients often complain of their joint pain, first manifesting more severely, in their shoulders and cervical (upper) spine area. These are the joints that are closest to the thyroid. Over time, these joint pains can spread to the other areas of the body, sometimes all the way down to the feet and all the way out to the fingertips.

Inflammation also tends to lead to stiffness in the joints as well, due to mild swelling and fluid around the joints, caused by the release of histamines that are also sent out by the immune system, that act as agents to overwhelm bacterial and viral intruders and reduce inflammation.

Patients with autoimmune thyroid disease, should closely monitor their joint symptoms once on treatment for their hypothyroidism because if they have joint symptoms that result in significant swelling, redness or pain that is more than mild to moderate, this could indicate the onset of Rheumatoid Arthritis (RA), another autoimmune disease, that affects the joints.

There are blood tests that help diagnose or rule out RA specifically, the main one being called "Rheumatoid Factor".

Two others that are sometimes also used in addition to RA Factor are the "ESR" (Erythrocyte Sedimentation Rate), which checks for high levels of inflammation in the body and the "ANA" (Anti-Nuclear Antibodies), which tests for systemic autoimmune disease activity.

One sign a patient can look for their self, is significant swelling and redness in a joint such as a hand, elbow, knee, etc... that is affected equally on both sides of the body. In other words, with Rheumatoid Arthritis, this will manifest in both joints simultaneously, on both sides of the body (symmetrically). Unfortunately, having one autoimmune disease, such as Hashimoto's, places a patient at a higher risk for developing other autoimmune disorders and is why this joint pain aspect should be monitored closely if rheumatic symptoms are occurring.

The mild to moderate muscle pain (rheumatic or fibromyalgic pain), in hypothyroidism which can include cramping and spasms, in my belief, is due to a slowing down of all organs in the body, due to lack of thyroid hormone, which also regulates our metabolism. This causes blood circulation to become less adequate and so the muscles are not nourished by blood and oxygen as they should be.

Strangely, some hypothyroid patients experience hypertension (high blood pressure) because the disease causes blood vessels to constrict but at the same time, they do not have proper blood circulation to some of their muscles because heart function is slightly reduced due to slowed metabolism.

This affect, also causes symptoms in tendons and ligaments and many hypothyroid patients also complain of "Carpal Tunnel Syndrome" (hand/wrist) and "Tarsal Tunnel Syndrome" (feet).

If a patient has severe, ongoing muscle symptoms, they should seek further medical testing, as I also recommended for joint pain patients, to rule out possible Muscle Disease and Connective Tissue Diseases. Some of the same tests as mentioned above are used to help diagnose muscle disease but there are others as well, such as one called "Anti-Smooth Muscle Antibodies". There are many Connective Tissue Diseases, including "Lupus" and some patients can experience "Overlap Syndromes", meaning they are experiencing more than one type.

A well-informed doctor is important when you are being treated for autoimmune hypothyroidism, one who understands the risks for other autoimmune disease disorders and one who can detect when symptoms may indicate something other than thyroid related ones. I have visited a few doctors in the past who actually did not know that hypothyroidism caused joint and muscle pain.

I have also known of other doctors who did not recognize emotional symptoms as being thyroid related in patients they were treating but actually believe these were separate issues. This is why a truly good, caring, well informed doctor is worth her/his weight in gold!

In conclusion I would like to add that many times, these mild to moderate joint pain symptoms, can be treated with over-the-counter anti-inflammatory medications.

There are also very effective over-the-counter, natural supplements that help with joint pain and inflammation, one of these being a combination of "Glucosamine and Chondroitin". It is also very important to take your thyroid medication as recommended by your Physician and let him/her know about other supplements you may choose to take in addition to your hormone replacement.

If it takes a prescription strength medication to treat your joint/muscle pain symptoms, it might be time to ask your doctor for further testing.

CHAPTER SIX

Fatigue Despite Thyroid Hormone Therapy?

The first thing I always suggest to treated hypothyroid patients who experience low energy and fatigue that is an important consideration when being replaced with thyroid hormone, is making sure the hormone therapy is being as optimized as possible.

Some doctors only treat to get the TSH level anywhere within the normal range but some patients need a TSH that is really suppressed, in order to feel better. The low normal at most labs for TSH is from about 0.3 to 0.5 and some patients need theirs to be at these lowest normal levels to see significant symptom relief and a doctor willing to work with them in trials of doses that get them there.

If you haven't received copies of labs you've had done to monitor your thyroid hormone therapy, I would ask for your most recent ones, to see where your doctor has put your TSH level (the "HIPPA" law in the U.S. grants patient's copies). If he has kept your TSH level at above 2.0 especially, you need to discuss a trial of a dose that will suppress the level down to below a 1.0 or even lower-normal.

Some doctors are overly concerned that getting TSH that low will cause hyperthyroid symptoms however this won't happen with close monitoring and with also testing the Free T-3 and Free T-4 levels for better monitoring of a dose that suppresses your TSH.

Other than this, I like to suggest a good multi-vitamin to thyroid patients but especially ones with B-12 and the other B vitamins because these help with energy. The sublingual type (liquid, i.e. "Perfect B" Brand) is good because it absorbs quickly and can be taken twice daily to help maintain energy levels through the day.

Some patients also report better symptom relief and improved energy levels by cutting wheat and dairy from their diet as well (takes discipline). This is due to the fact that glutton intolerance (sensitivity to wheat products) is more common in autoimmune thyroid patients and dairy products can flare the symptoms of lactose intolerance in thyroid patients as well. Both conditions have potential to negatively affect energy levels in the body.

These are suggestions that can aid thyroid hormone therapy in relieving hypothyroid symptoms, including low energy and fatigue, the best possible.

CHAPTER SEVEN

Is Dysautonomia Common in Thyroid Patients?

"Dysautonoma", is one of those disorders that is similar in
recognition to CFS, Fibromyalgia and adrenal fatigue,
being a disorder that comes in several types, that like these
others is not known about or recognized by many Doctors,
although it is gaining recognition. There are a very real
group of disorders that are in the dysautonomia category,
recognized and described in detail, on the most reputable
medical sources, including the National Institutes of
Health.

Dysautonomia disorders cause dysfunction of the
involuntary nervous system at different levels of severity,
also called the "autonomic nervous system". This is the
part of our nervous system that regulates involuntary
bodily functions such as heart rate, respiration, liver
function, kidney function, adrenal function, etc…. Some of
these functions you might think we control but actually we
can only influence them because when you sleep, heart
beat and breathing continues, as do these other involuntary
bodily functions.

Some types of dysautonomia, are more commonly found in
thyroid patients, such as Mitral Valve Prolapse Syndrome
(some medical sites add "dysautonomia" into the MVPS
title). While the Mitral ValveProlapse itself, is a heart
murmur, caused by looseness or thickness of the mitral
valve leaflets in the heart, many reputable medical sources
state that people who actually have symptoms from it,
have a co-morbid dysautonomia with it.

They actually do not know if MVP causes dysautonomia in some patients or if the co-existence of dysautonomia with MVP is what causes more symptoms (syndrome). I personally believe the latter theory is the one that is more likely.

Another very common form of dysautonomia is "orthostatic hypotension", also referred to as "postural hypotention". This one causes you to feel faint, due to a blood pressure drop upon standing from a seated or lying down position (supine positions) and it is also sometimes referred to as "neurally mediated hypotension" (NMH). This form of dysautonomia is also found in conditions such as CFS, Fibromyalgia and conditions that affect adrenal function. They also do not know if this type dysautonomia, with broader aspects to it, is the cause of these syndromes or just part of the manifestations of them.

There is a medical test for this one, called the "tilt-table test", which consists of taking a patient's blood pressure and heart rate readings, when sitting or lying flat, then again when at various upright positions. I have this type of dysautonomia and would be revealed clearly if I were to have this tilt-table test done. You can do a home-version of this test yourself using a BP monitor, by first taking a reading while sitting, then again immediately upon standing to monitor for abnormal changes.

When I do this test at home, my BP drops a good 20 points and my heart rate increases 30 or more BPM. This is too much of a fluctuation and an overreaction by the involuntary nervous system.

This would also be revealed via a tilt-table test and points to an involuntary nervous system that is struggling to regulate these bodily functions (dysregulated-autonomic "dys-autonomia").

The treatment for OH is usually simple lifestyle changes, when it is mild to moderate, including exercise and eating healthy, making sure there is ample salt in the diet and drinking plenty of water which all help to keep low blood pressure episodes from happening (hypotension). When drug therapy for OH is used, it may include "Fludrocortisone" (Florinef), a mineral corticosteroid used to help regulate blood pressure, Midodrine (alpha-1 adrenergic agonist), Methylphenidate (amphetamine) and Ephedrine (adrenaline). These drug treatments are not recommended or prescribed however, when lifestyle and diet changes are able to control OH.

I have had this form of dysautonomia, since childhood but much worse since experiencing the onset of autoimmune thyroid disease. Interestingly, I was also diagnosed with a heart murmur, at age 14 or 15 and an MD and a Cardiologist, both thought it was "Wolf-Parkinson-White Syndrome" (a more serious heart murmur) but a modern-day cardiologist ruled it out and I now know they were detecting MVP in me because much less was know about it and dysautonomia in the 1970s.

If a patient suspects they have a form of dysautonomia, they should discuss this with their Doctor. The patient might then be referred to a specialist who is familiar with the group of disorders that come under this heading.

These include; Postural Orthostatic Tachycardia Syndrome (POTS), Neurocardiogenic Syncope, Mitral Valve Prolapse Dysautonomia, Pure Autonomic Failure, Multiple System Atrophy (Shy-Drager syndrome), Autonomic Instability and other less severe types including Orthostatic Hypotension, which can manifest alone or as a feature of one of these others or syndromes that may also include it as a feature.

Dysautonomia can be a mild condition or severe and even life-threatening and so it is important that patients, who suspect they have it, are diagnosed and treated.

CHAPTER EIGHT

Anxiety, Panic and Depression

If you have thyroid disease, you may have experienced some co-morbid (related) anxiety along with it. This can especially be true if you have autoimmune thyroid disease, which includes Graves' Disease/hyperthyroidism and Hashimoto's thyroiditis, which can cause Hashitoxicosis (intermittent hyperthyroidism).

A very unpleasant type of anxiety reaction is one called "panic attacks" and if you experience them frequently, it is referred to as "Panic Disorder". These are very unpleasant anxiety attacks that cause anxiety symptoms to escalate suddenly.

When people experience them, they will often hyperventilate and experience a racing heart and an extreme fear emotion. This article is intended to show you that you are far from being alone in experiencing these.

Panic Disorder Description and Statistics

"Panic Attacks" are what you might describe as the "climax of anxiety" and are truly unpleasant, to say the least, as we who have experienced them know!

They can occur with just about any other anxiety disorder, including Generalized Anxiety Disorder (GAD) but when the panic attacks themselves are the feature-manifestation, it is referred to as "Panic Disorder" (PD). They can hit extremely hard and a person first experiencing them will commonly believe they are having a heart attack.

Many people new to the panic attack experience find their selves in hospital emergency rooms, only to be told everything physically checks out normal, once they return to a calmed state. Many new to the panic experience will also believe they are going mad/insane or that another attack will cause them to completely lose control.

Approximately 6 million American adults ages 18 and older, or about 2.7 percent of people in this age group in a given year, have panic disorder. Panic disorder typically develops in early adulthood (median age of onset is 24), but the age of onset extends throughout adulthood. About one in three people with panic disorder develops agoraphobia, a condition in which the individual becomes afraid of being in any place or situation where escape might be difficult or help unavailable in the event of a panic attack (statistics by the National Institute of Mental Health, reprints allowed for public education).

Hypothyroid Therapy and Anxiety/Depression

What is really important when a thyroid patient is being treated for hypothyroidism is that they are on optimal dose of "thyroid hormone replacement therapy medication" (HRT). When a patient is placed on a dose of HRT, most will need 1, 2 or 3 dose changes (usually increases) before they reach the adequate/optimal level.

When some Doctors place a patient on thyroid hormone and if that first dose gets their thyroid blood lab levels, anywhere into the normal range, they simply stop there. They do not afterward try to "optimize" the patient's HRT.

Some patients need more of a targeted treatment goal, for example, many patients do not see symptoms resolve significantly, unless their dose gets their "TSH" level (most common thyroid lab test Doctors use to monitor HRT), at about "1.0" and some may even need their TSH level at lowest normal, which is about "0.3 to 0.5". A Doctor has to be willing to work with a patient in getting their HRT optimized, by going by their symptoms as well as their lab levels.

In regard to emotional symptoms caused by thyroid disease, anxiety and depression are commonly listed and patients not being treated optimally may see these symptoms linger. Some do also need the addition of antidepressant and anti-anxiety medications but some patients see their emotional symptoms resolve with thyroid HRT alone.

In my case as a hypothyroid patient, once I was treated on the correct dose of thyroid HRT, my emotional symptoms of anxiety and depression resolved within a couple of months. Previous to this however, I was treated by a different doctor who did not optimize my HRT and I struggled with anxiety and depressive symptoms for nearly two years. That doctor kept my TSH between 3.0 and 5.0 and I'm the type patient that needs a very low TSH (lowest normal). Not all patients need a lowest-normal TSH to see symptom relief but a good target range to start with, is the "1.0" I mention above.

Some Doctors will claim that depression and anxiety are not caused by hypothyroidism but it certainly is, especially the autoimmune type-Hashimoto's (type I have) and many research studies have concluded this.

Almost all reputable medical sources list "depression" as a symptom of hypothyroidism and many have added "anxiety" to the list as well.

Patients should be pro-active in discussing optimal HRT with their Doctors because it is after all a person's health at stake, which affects every aspect of their lives. It is only right that hypothyroid patients be treated, so that they can pursue their livelihood, family needs and enjoyment and all around quality of life.

There are sensational Doctors out there but the ones, who don't understand the need to optimally treat hypothyroid patients, in my opinion, should refer their hypothyroid patients, to the Doctors who do believe in thyroid HRT optimization.

CHAPTER NINE

Metabolic Related Complications

Hypothyroidism and Fatty Liver Disease

As I mention in other articles, people with one metabolic disorder, including thyroid disease, are at higher risk for developing other metabolic disorders and diseases. For example, a patient with hypothyroidism is at increased risk for developing Metabolic Syndrome (a pre-diabetes syndrome), Adult Onset Diabetes and Adrenal Syndromes/Diseases. This is especially true if the thyroid disease they have is the autoimmune type.

Another metabolic related condition that can occur in thyroid patients, as well as in a large percent of the population is one called "Non-Alcoholic Fatty Liver Disease" (NAFLD). This disease is metabolic related due to the fact that the body is storing an excessive amount of fat in this major organ called the liver, rather than converting more of it into energy needed by the body. One reason this happens is due to over-consumption of fats and sugars, combined with being overweight and the inability of the liver to keep up with the demand for conversion of these into energy.

When the liver becomes overwhelmed in this performance of duty, it instead begins to store more fat. Over time, this causes mild inflammation in the liver and liver cell damage (hepatic response or "steatosis hepatitis") and over time can actually cause lesions in the liver or "liver sclerosis".

While most cases of fatty liver do not lead to actual hepatitis or sclerosis, it is a risk people with fatty liver should be aware of, so that they can undertake diet and lifestyle changes, in order to keep the condition under control and to possibly resolve or reverse it over time.

Most cases of fatty liver disease are caused by alcohol consumption and since this type I'm addressing in this article is not, the "non-alcoholic" prefix is used. It is true however that despite the fact it is not alcohol related, people with the non-alcoholic type are highly advised to avoid alcohol consumption.

What are some other ways to help control and possibly resolve NAFLD that some statistics state may affect up to one-third of the population? Well, as is recommended for most metabolic disorders and diseases, patients need to incorporate a healthy regimen of exercise and weight loss/control into their schedules. Even if this means simply walking for 20 minutes at least three times per week.

Patients should also avoid fatty foods and refined sugars which both can be stored as fat in the liver. Eating more fruits and vegetables and foods containing lots of fiber can also help with this disease. It is also important to lose weight when you are carrying extra pounds, especially that that accumulates in the mid-section of the body.

Most people have no physical symptoms of this disease although the most common symptoms reported are fatigue and dull pain on the right side, just under the rib cage. NAFLD is usually found incidentally when a patient is blood tested and the tests include a metabolic panel that includes liver function tests.

Their liver enzymes will be mildly to moderately, elevated (ALT and SGPT or AST levels). Once these abnormal liver counts are found, an ultrasound imaging of the liver is performed to confirm fatty infiltration of the liver.

If you are a thyroid disease patient, or one that has Metabolic Syndrome or Diabetes, a "Metabolic Panel" including liver function tests should be performed via blood testing, once a year, to detect possible development of fatty liver disease. If this disorder is detected a Doctor may prescribe a treatment plan similar to the one I describe above but medications may also be prescribed in more severe cases.

Hypothyroidism and Metabolic Syndrome

There are many co-morbid disorders that can affect thyroid patients. One of those is a syndrome affecting the body's metabolism, called "Metabolic Syndrome". According to reputable medical sources, this syndrome affects millions of people and puts them at higher risk for developing diabetes, heart disease and other potentially serious health problems.

This syndrome has gained recognition because of its ability to significantly increase the risk for diabetes and in past years was known by other names including "Syndrome X".

Medical research conclusions link the Metabolic Syndrome to thyroid dysfunction, some including the link listed below (type into your PC browser to view), associate it with "sub-clinical hypothyroidism".

What I feel is significant about this study is the fact that most hypothyroid patients who are later treated, experienced long standing sub-clinical hypothyroidism, before progressing to overt (full blown) hypothyroidism. This means most of us who were diagnosed with hypothyroidism, were at risk for Metabolic Syndrome.

Link>
http://jcem.endojournals.org/cgi/content/abstract/jc.2006-1718v1 (Journal of Clinical Endocrinology & Metabolism)

Metabolic Syndrome occurs when a person gains extra weight and has become less active, so that their bodies lack the needed exercise to help them burn fat and calories. The hormone in the body that aids in this process is "insulin". This pancreatic hormone takes glucose, fats and carbohydrates (sugar, starch, cellulose) and helps to convert them into energy that is needed by the body. Glucose is essential in the body and without it, the body cannot function.

A major organ that depends highly upon glucose is the brain. When someone who is at risk for developing Metabolic Syndrome due to being overweight and inactive consumes fats, sugars and carbohydrates, their bodies begin to store these rather than burn them off or convert them into energy. The lack of glucose metabolism is referred to as "Insulin Resistance".

Over time, insulin resistance can evolve into Type II Diabetes or what is also referred to as Adult Onset Diabetes. In addition to this syndrome increasing the risk of diabetes, it can also contribute to hypertension, elevated cholesterol and heart disease.

Other medical sources also associate Metabolic Syndrome with Non-Alcoholic Fatty Liver Disease (NAFLD).

The symptoms that indicate development of this syndrome include; weight gain, especially in the mid-section of your body, development of hypertension, hypoglycemic episodes (lows in glucose energy levels before and after meals), mood swings and inability to concentrate (brain fog). People, who are developing this disorder, will often have borderline diabetic glucose levels, when they are blood lab tested for diabetes. They will also often have elevated cholesterol and triglyceride levels.

Improving your diet by eliminating refined sugars, cutting back on unhealthy fats (saturated/trans fats) and simple carbohydrates (pies, cakes, candies & soft drinks) and eating more complex carbohydrates (fruits vegetables, nuts & grains) plus keeping your weight down and exercising will significantly reduce your chances of developing Metabolic Syndrome and the serious health complications that can develop from it.

Thyroid patients with hypothyroidism are at increased risk for other metabolic disorders, such as diabetes as well as this pre-diabetes condition called Metabolic Syndrome.

Preventing Diabetes in Thyroid Patients

Type 2 Diabetes is also called Adult Onset Diabetes and affects an estimated 15-million Americans. It is more common in adults ages 45 and over and more common in people with other endocrine disorders, including thyroid diseases.

There are steps that can be taken to reduce your risk of experiencing the onset of this disease that causes a dysfunction in the way your body metabolizes your blood sugar (glucose), as outlined below.

Avoid weight gain and excessively high blood glucose, by being faithful to a diet low in refined sugars. Refined sugars are those that do not come naturally but are processed sugars used to manufacture junk foods, such as cakes, cookies, candies, pies and soft drinks. Consuming too much refined sugar not only causes excess weight gain but over time, can also cause the body to lose its ability to regulate that sugar via the hormone called insulin.

This hormone that is released by the pancreas, helps metabolize (convert) the sugar we consume, into energy for the body and helps carry that energy to every cell in the body.

Without adequate glucose in the blood, our organs do not function properly and one major organ that is highly dependent upon glucose is the brain as previously mentioned. There is however a limit to how much glucose the body is able to metabolize and when there is a continual excess of it, it is converted into fat and carbohydrates as well and stored in the body.

Over time, this causes weight gain and an inability of the body to continue converting the excess amounts of glucose being consumed and at this point, a person may develop a condition called "insulin resistance", a pre-diabetic condition that over time has the potential to become full blown diabetes.

Incorporate adequate exercise into your weekly schedule, which helps to keep your weight down and helps the body to metabolize glucose. Exercise is essential in helping to burn calories and fat in the body, so that less of it is stored. Exercise also helps the body to build muscle tissue from the things we eat, rather than inactivity, which contributes to the body storing more fat. It also helps the body by circulating the hormones that are active in the blood stream and that contribute to our health, energy and metabolism, including insulin, which regulates our blood glucose levels. Even mild exercise such as walking for 20 minutes, three or more times a week, can help the body with metabolism and prevention of weight gain and can contribute to weight loss.

Get regular check ups by your Doctor and monitor your glucose levels regularly, especially if diabetes runs in your family. It is a good idea for everyone to get yearly check ups by their Doctor but if one or both of your parents or one of your siblings has diabetes, this becomes even more important. Diabetes, like other endocrine diseases (glandular), can run in families and so if a close relative has diabetes, you are at significantly increased risk for developing the disease yourself.

Early prevention is the key to avoiding this potentially serious disease, which upon experiencing the onset of, also puts a person at higher risk for heart disease, kidney failure and glaucoma, which is an eye disorder that can eventually lead to diminished eyesight and even blindness.

Home glucose monitors are available, that allow a person to check their own blood glucose levels regularly, in the convenience of their home.

A person at risk for diabetes can check their glucose level at different times of the day and keep a record of their readings, so that they can detect any pattern or change in their glucose regulation and report these changes to their Doctor.

Avoid alcohol or only consume it in cautious moderation. People at risk for diabetes or who actually have diabetes are cautioned to avoid alcohol if possible or to at least drink it in moderation. Alcohol reacts very quickly in the body and your body depends on your liver to clear the alcohol from your system because it is recognized by the body as a toxin. When you drink alcohol, the liver will not function in converting glucose into carbohydrates and fat because it is busy clearing the body of alcohol and this, results in a spike or increase in glucose levels in the blood.

People who are on insulin shots to treat their diabetes or on an oral medication can seriously hinder the effectiveness of their medication, through alcohol consumption and this is especially true when they consume alcohol on an empty stomach or in excessive amounts.

The liver and the hormone insulin, both work in the body to regulate glucose, the liver being the organ that converts it into fat and carbohydrates or "stored energy" and insulin being the hormone that converts it into "immediate energy" for the cells of the body.

Treated Hypothyroidism and Weight Gain

It is a well known fact that untreated hypothyroidism causes moderate weight gain, in fact some patients report weight gain that is in excess of moderate.

I use the term moderate however, because most medical sources state it that way and they also suggest that weight gain with untreated hypothyroidism will usually result in no more than 20lb of weight gain.

Regardless of the actual amount of weight gain, which in my opinion varies among individual patients and depends upon how severe their untreated hypothyroidism is, it does indeed cause weight gain! This is due to the fact that with hypothyroid conditions, the rate of our bodily metabolism is slowed down. We burn less energy when the metabolism is not running at a normal rate. They also refer to this as hypo-metabolism, which can have additional causes other than hypothyroidism.

Now when we look at patients who are being treated for hypothyroidism, we still hear them report gaining weight more easily and having difficulty losing weight. There are no medical research studies on the subject of weight gain in patients being treated for hypothyroidism that I am aware of but the number of patients attesting to this problem in articles and on forums is significant. I personally can also attest to the fact that I too gain weight more easily and have a harder time losing weight, despite being adequately and even optimally treated for my hypothyroidism.

I'm not sure we will ever have a firm medical explanation as to why this happens but it could possibly be that thyroid hormone being administered from the outside (hormone therapy), whether it is the natural or synthetic form, is slightly less effective in regulating our metabolism than our own hormone is.

This is certainly just a theory but in my opinion, is a reasonable one that should be given some consideration by those in the medical profession.

Another theory that I believe should be considered, is the possibility that "thyroid autoimmunity" that is present in most cases of hypothyroidism, may also play a factor in weight control. It may be that thyroid antibodies also affect our metabolism, to a very small degree but significant enough to affect our body's ability to burn calories and turn fat into energy. I do know that "insulin resistance" is more common in treated hypothyroid patients and the description I just gave, fits this condition. I can also attest to being a hypothyroid patient with co-morbid insulin resistance.

Treated hypothyroid patients must work harder than people without thyroid disease, to lose weight and to keep their weight under control. While there are many diet plans out there, I feel the same principles apply in weight loss, no matter which diet plan you may try.

The principles include eating healthier, which would consist of eating more fruits, vegetables, nuts and grains, cutting back and eliminating refined sugars from your diet, eating less and exercising more. These principles can be wrapped together in many different packages and called by many different diet-plan names but they are the principles that work and you simply add discipline to that plan, to make it work.

Weight gain and difficulty losing weight is a challenge to treated hypothyroid patients but one they can accomplish with effort.

CHAPTER TEN

Thyroid Eye Disease

Graves' Ophthalmology (GO) is a co-occurring inflammatory condition affecting the eyes (also called Thyroid Eye Disease). Some medical sources state that GO is present to varied degrees in 50% of Graves' disease patients (those with autoimmune hyperthyroidism) but only requires corrective surgical procedures in approximately 5% of cases.

This means it can potentially develop in up to half of Grave's patients and rarely a type of this condition can also develop in patients with Hashimoto's thyroiditis (in about 2% of patients with autoimmune hypothyroidism). It can also cause bulging of the eyes (proptosis) and possible deterioration of vision. The duration of symptoms can occur for 1 to 3 years before they resolve through the natural course of the disease and/or through treatments, if necessary and depending on the severity of its manifestation.

The most common treatments for GO/Thyroid Eye Disease include:

• *Eye drops to keep the eyes lubricated*

• *Corticosteroid therapy (steroid anti-inflammatory)*

• *Radiotherapy and/or Decompression Therapy to reduce orbital damage*

• *Eyelid surgery to lengthen eyelids that may not cover the eyes well due to them bulging ---*

• GD patients who smoke are sometimes also given the recommendation by their doctors to quit smoking because of the inflammatory chemicals contained in cigarettes that can potentially affect the eyes.

(TED) can cause serious damage and even blindness in some patients. Unfortunately, with regard to Graves ' disease, patients who do develop Graves' Ophthalmology (GO), treatment for the condition may not be able to prevent eye damage even though they are already well treated for their hyperthyroidism.

CHAPTER ELEVEN

Adrenal Fatigue and Thyroid Patients

A lot of us with thyroid disease also have some co-existing adrenal fatigue and in fact have been discussing this quite a bit on some of the thyroid forums and message boards for a number of years.

Add to thyroid disease, something like a traumatic or very stressful even and you can really suffer from adrenal fatigue. Your circadian rhythms are off with this condition and are why your sleep patterns are disrupted. Your cortisol and DHEA will have their peaks, at the wrong times, such as at sleep time and your normal drop in these hormones also happens at the wrong time, like during the day, when you most need the peak energy. Adrenal fatigue that goes on for a long time (chronic) then becomes "adrenal exhaustion" and this is the point to where you no longer experience those needed peak levels at all.

I have had adrenal fatigue for several years, as a feature of Chronic Fatigue Syndrome and have also experienced adrenal exhaustion. Mine turned into adrenal exhaustion, after experiencing the onset of Hashimoto's/hypothyroidism and at the same time, I had gone through a terribly stressful period of time (chronic stressors).

Mine did not improve when I first began thyroid hormone replacement but actually worsened for a time. After several months on the correct thyroid dose, I finally saw some improvement in thyroid and adrenal symptoms.

However, at times of extra stress and extended periods of hard physical activity, I've taken some adrenal support supplements that I learned about when researching about adrenal fatigue. These included multi "B" vitamins, especially B-12, in sublingual form (liquid) and vitamin "C", magnesium, selenium, zinc, DHEA 25mg (an over-the-counter adrenal hormone) and sometimes but less often, an Adrenal Cortex Extract (processed beef adrenal glands in pill form).

These always help me a great deal but I don't supplement with the ones containing actual adrenal hormone, as a permanent regimen but as safe as they are at the recommended doses, it would not hurt for me to do so, according to research that has been conducted on these supplements.

I seriously considered Cortef (natural adrenal steroid) and had a Dr. willing to treat me with it but I was just a little wary of steroids and I still am. I have however, read many reputable medical resources that state that Cortef is safe as physiological doses (25mg and less), to supplement a person's low cortisol levels from adrenal exhaustion but can cause "adrenal suppression", if administered in full replacement doses (above 25mg) and if used for extended periods. In my opinion, adrenal support supplements are usually all that is needed for most cases of adrenal fatigue.

How does a patient know if they have adrenal fatigue? Blood adrenal hormone levels can be helpful but are like a "snapshot reading" and since cortisol levels go up when you are stressed, like at a blood draw, this can affect the snapshot blood level.

112

This is why saliva testing is recommended because you can conveniently get several readings over a 24 hour period to establish the adrenal hormone rhythms.

Saliva testing has been researched and found very accurate, in fact it is used to monitor hormone levels in medical research, including that done by the World Health Organizations. It is also an approved form of testing, by many major health insurance companies, such as Blue Cross/Blue Shield.

Many pharmacies carry the type manufactured by "ZRT Labs, Inc.", which is also a U.S. approved blood lab, so you might check with your pharmacy to see if they carry this brand, if you suspect adrenal fatigue is affecting you.

Most adrenal saliva tests are not really expensive and can be diagnostic in detecting adrenal fatigue.

While the above list of thyroid disease complications does not include all of them, these are some of the major ones that are experienced. If you suspect you are experiencing a complication of thyroid disease or a co-morbid condition, see your doctor for further evaluation and treatment options.

CHAPTER TWELVE

What are Goiters?

When a thyroid patient has a goiter, this simply means they have swelling of the thyroid gland, which is located at the front of the neck, in the area just below the Adam's apple. Goiters are recognized as different types and as affecting part of the thyroid, such as one of the two lobes (one on each side of the gland) or the middle part of the gland called the isthmus or as affecting the entire gland as a whole. They are also considered different types depending upon the causes of them.

How Goiters are Detected/Diagnosed

Patients, who have goiters or are suspected of having them, may be referred for a "thyroid ultrasound" (sound-wave imaging/sonogram) or "thyroid uptake scan" (radiology/radioactive iodine) and possibly even an MRI (Magnetic Resonance Imaging). These are diagnostic tests that give detailed images of the thyroid gland, to determine the size of goiters and whether they contain nodules within them that are not detectable by palpation.

Types of Goiters

A major cause of goiters, are autoimmune thyroid diseases. If a person's thyroid gland has swelling plus a number of small tumors called "nodules" within it, they refer to this type as a "multi-nodular goiter". The nodules within a gland that has goiter can be the type that causes the thyroid gland to produce excess thyroid hormone.

In this case, they will add the term "toxic" to the term, calling it a "toxic multi-nodular goiter".

People with Hashimoto's thyroiditis, commonly have multi-nodular goiters that are non- toxic. When a person is termed as having a "diffuse goiter", this means there is general swelling throughout the gland that is not caused by nodules. This type of goiter can also cause toxicity or over-activity of the thyroid gland (hyperthyroidism), in which case it is referred to as a "toxic diffuse goiter". These types are found commonly in patients with Grave's Disease, as well as toxic multi-nodular goiters.

If a goiter is caused by iodine deficiency, it is referred to as a "colloid nodular" or "endemic' goiter. This type is rare in the U.S. and many other industrialized countries that use iodized table salt, which usually provides those that consume it, enough iodine to avoid iodine deficiency hypothyroidism and the resulting endemic goiters.

Temporary types of thyroiditis, such as those that occur with viral infections and in pregnant women can also cause goiter (asymmetrical enlargement) but these type will resolve within a few weeks, along with the thyroiditis. These type goiters can flare up short term with these types of thyroiditis and cause severe pain in the thyroid gland, which is referred to as "sub-acute thyroiditis", while others types do not cause a painful thyroid which is referred to as "silent thyroiditis".

CHAPTER THIRTEEN

What are Thyroid Nodules?

Thyroid nodules are small tumor-like growths on the thyroid gland. According to statistics, as much as 10 percent of the population has thyroid nodules but they occur far more often in thyroid diseases. People with autoimmune thyroid diseases have abnormal thyroid tissue and over time can develop a large number of nodules or what is referred to as "multi-nodules".

How Thyroid Nodules are Detected/Diagnosed

Thyroid nodules can be detected by feel or "palpation" but some may be in an area of the gland that are only detectable by diagnostic imaging tests such as "thyroid ultrasound" (sound wave imaging), "Radio Active Iodine Uptake Scans" (radiological imaging) and "MRI" (Magnetic Resonance Imaging).

Thyroid nodules that are solitary or found to be a single one, rather than found among a group of them have a slightly higher risk of containing cancer cells (malignancy) than do multi-nodules and larger nodules are also considered more suspicious. When a solitary nodule is located, the treating Doctor may wish to have a tissue biopsy performed.

The procedure that is usually performed to obtain a thyroid nodule tissue sample is called a "Fine Needle Aspiration" (FNA) and is a simple out-patient procedure.

The tissue sample is then lab-analyzed to detect any abnormal cells indicating the presence of either "papillary" or "follicular" cancer, which are the two major types that can potentially invade the thyroid gland.

Types of Thyroid Nodules

When thyroid nodules are being investigated, they may be placed into several categories. Two of the more basic categories of thyroid nodules, are those that are solitary (single ones) and multi-nodules (a group of several) but other terms used in describing them include "hot nodules", meaning the nodule is actively absorbing iodine from the thyroid gland and is releasing thyroid hormone, causing a hormone imbalance in the patient (hyperthyroidism).

Smaller hot nodules may not cause hyperthyroidism while larger ones usually do and many times are also biopsied due to their larger size. If the nodule is not causing thyroid hormone release, it is referred to as a "cold nodule" and both hot and cold nodules have a distinct appearance on diagnostic imaging tests.

Some thyroid nodules are more solid than others which are referred to as a "solid nodules" and these are also considered more suspicious of possibly containing cancer cells and may also be biopsied as a precaution, depending upon their size. Many non-solid nodules are considered to be "cystic nodules" because they will contain fluid in the center of them and these type, are almost never considered a risk for containing cancer cells.

Treatment for Goiters and Thyroid Nodules

The most common treatment for both goiters and benign thyroid nodules is thyroid hormone replacement therapy. Treating doctors will prescribe a dose of thyroid hormone that can help to shrink goiters and nodules over time and can also prevent further growth of them.

If a goiter or thyroid nodule is large enough to obstruct a patient's breathing or swallowing, a treating doctor might refer the patient for surgery, to remove a nodule or part of the thyroid gland and possibly all of the thyroid gland.

In cases of malignancy found in the thyroid gland, total thyroid removal is always the treatment. Afterward the patient must have thyroid hormone replacement therapy for the rest of their lives. More in regard to malignant thyroid conditions will be discussed in the next segments addressing thyroid cancer.

CHAPTER FOURTEEN

Hashimoto's Encephalopathy Rare but Serious

There is a neuro-endocrine disorder that causes very
serious and potentially life threatening symptoms, called
Hashimoto's Encephalopathy (HE). The disorder can occur
in patients with Hashimoto'sthyroiditis, who experience a
very high elevation of "thyroid antibody" levels. These
antibodies, that attack the thyroid gland after recognition
of it by the immune system, as a foreign invader, can
become highly elevated in these rare cases of HE. At these
high elevations they will begin to affect brain and nerve
function in the body or the "neurological system". Severe
symptoms will result because this system is the body's
information and communication center and a disruption
from a disease process can cause an array of nerve and
brain related symptoms.

Inflammation caused by the antibodies (also called auto-
antibodies) spreads to the brain and begins to affect the
tissue containing the nerves that control bodily functions
and impulses throughout the body. The resulting effect, are
severe neurological symptoms, meaning abnormal
responses and manifestations of nervous system
dysfunction.

These symptoms can include; psychotic episodes
(hallucinations and delusions, dementia (mental
deterioration), neuropathies (abnormal nerve sensations)
and even coma or death if left untreated.

The antibodies responsible for causing thyroid destruction and inflammation in the thyroid gland but that can also cause HE when highly elevated, are the "TPO" (anti-thyroidperoxidase) and "TG" (anti-thyroglobulin) antibodies. This autoimmune process, called Hashimoto's thyroiditis that can result in the less common Hashimoto's Encephalopathy, is more often a result of elevated anti-TPO levels although it can result from elevations of both it and the anti-TG antibodies.

Thyroid hormone levels are not usually a factor in this potentially serious neuro-endocrine disorder of thyroid autoimmunity. Some patients in fact have been documented in medical research, to have experienced HE with their thyroid hormone levels in normal range and before they were in need of thyroid hormone replacement therapy. This disorder is a rare but a strong example of the fact that thyroid antibodies have the ability to produce bodily symptoms regardless of thyroid hormone levels.

Treatment for HE, is to reduce the inflammation caused by the thyroid antibodies by administering a steroid anti-inflammatory drug to patients who are diagnosed. These drugs, also called corticosteroids or hydrocortisone, mimic the anti-inflammatory properties of our body's own natural anti-inflammatory called "cortisol".

A major brand prescribed for inflammatory conditions is "Prednisone", a powerful steroid that usually achieves an anti-inflammatory effect quickly with only a relatively short term regimen being necessary to correct cases of HE.

If a patient with Hashimoto's thyroiditis or their loved ones, notice the onset of sudden and severe neurological symptoms, they should report to their Doctor immediately, to rule out HE as the cause. A delay in treatment for a patient experiencing this very rare disorder could result in severe consequences.

It is my sincere hope that I have helped to provide a general understanding to the readers of this book, in regard to those complications that commonly, less-commonly and rarely occur with thyroid diseases and disorders.

(END - Section Three)

SECTION FOUR:

Neuropathy and Myopathy in Treated Thyroid Disease

(Hypothyroid and Hyperthyoid Nerve Pain and Muscle Weakness)

INTRODUCTION:

Thyroid disease patients can experience a number of different complications as a result of their hypothyroid (underactive thyroid) or hyperthyroid (overactive thyroid) conditions. Two of these complications are nerve pain and dysfunction, referred to as "peripheral neuropathy" and muscle weakness with possible atrophy (shrinkage of muscles), referred to as "thyroid myopathy".

In some cases, these two problems that are co-morbid to thyroid disorders can coexist, so that they are occurring at the same time and this may be referred to as "neuromuscular disease". This is a symptom-aspect that has less information available on it via online medical search, than do the more common thyroid-related problems, such as weight gain, joint pain and fatigue.

Within the chapters of this book, that follow, I hope to present to the reader, a general understanding of these often debilitating and potentially very serious manifestations of thyroid disease, affecting the nerves and muscles of the body, including the treatments available for them.

I present this information to you as a fellow hypothyroid patient with autoimmune thyroiditis and co-morbid peripheral neuropathy and myopathy, which inspired me to search and research the information contained in the chapters.

-*Jim Lowrance*

TABLE OF CONTENTS:

CHAPTER ONE

What Components of Thyroid Disease causes Neuropathy and/or Myopathy?

After reading much of the medical research that is available regarding peripheral neuropathy and myopathy that results from thyroid disease, I have come to the conclusion that these problems can potentially result from the autoimmune aspect of thyroid disease or from the metabolic aspect of it or as a result of both these components, simultaneously.

While myopathy is simply a term for muscle weakness that can include atrophy (muscle wasting), peripheral neuropathy is a term that includes sensory symptoms (i.e. burning, tingling and numbness), motor symptoms (i.e. muscle weakness and difficulty controlling movements in them) and autonomic symptoms (i.e. changes in involuntary body functions, such as digestion, sweating, cardiopulmonary and other organ functions). In some patients with nerve pain, only one limb or area of their body is affected (mono-neuropathy), while others see many areas of the body affected simultaneously (poly-neuropathy).

Autoimmune Hypothyroidism

The autoimmune aspect of thyroid disease that can be involved in the previously-described symptoms and others is the disease process that results in hormone imbalances of either the underactive or overactive thyroid types.

The underactive type, also referred to as "hypothyroidism", is often the result of auto-antibodies from the immune system, that mistakenly attack the thyroid gland, which is referred to as autoimmune thyroiditis.

The types of hypothyroid autoimmunity are somewhat varied but the most common type in industrialized countries is "Hashimoto's disease", also referred to as "chronic lymphocytic thyroiditis".

This common form of thyroiditis, results from the creation of auto-antibodies, from the immune system, that attack key thyroid proteins that are responsible for the manufacture of thyroid hormones, from iodine that enters the body via the diet.

These two key proteins are the "thyroid Peroxidase" and the "thyroglobulin" and when these are attacked and destroyed by auto-antibodies, they are referred to as the "anti-thyroidperoxidase" and "anti-thyroglobulin" antibodies (abbreviated on blood lab tests as "Anti-TPO" and anti-TG").

These eventually cause enough damage and destruction to the thyroid gland as to cause it to manufacture abnormally low levels of thyroid hormone, which reduces the speed of metabolism in the body. The purpose of these hormones is to regulate a proper level of metabolism -- the production of energy that results from things consumed into the body (i.e. food, water and oxygen).

Autoimmune Hyperthyroidism

In the case of autoimmune overactive thyroid gland disease, also referred to as "Graves' disease", the type of auto-antibodies that cause the opposite effect of abnormally high thyroid antibodies in the body, are called "thyroid stimulating immunoglobulin" (abbreviated "TSI"). These are sent from the immune system and attach to key proteins in the thyroid gland, causing them to become overly-stimulated in producing thyroid hormone from iodine.

Some medical sources state that the TSI antibody mimics the effects of a naturally occurring hormone sent from the pituitary brain-gland, called "thyroid stimulating hormone" (abbreviated "TSH"). The pituitary gland fluctuates in the level of this necessary hormone that it sends to the thyroid gland, to properly regulate the amount of thyroid hormones manufactured and dispersed throughout all the cells of the body. It does-so, by sensing how much of these hormones the body needs at any given time, the main ones being the "T4" (containing 4 iodine molecules) and the "T3" (containing 3 iodine molecules). It is a very sensitive system that adjusts to physical activity levels and other factors that require changes in bodily metabolism but it becomes disrupted when the thyroid gland is being attacked by either hypothyroid or hyperthyroid causing antibodies.

Autoimmunity of any kind is a strange thing. With autoimmune diseases, the body begins to attack itself for reasons that we simply have no understanding of at this stage.

This, despite there being significant numbers of medical research studies on the subject that have been published by medical groups for decades. For some reason, the immune system will begin to attack natural, normal tissues in the body, as if they are something that presents a danger to the rest of the body.

These specially-created antibodies are usually sent-out to destroy viruses and bacteria or to control allergens that might enter the body via airborne particles that are breathed-in or that are consumed in food or water.

When a part of the body that does not present a threat to us is attacked by this autoimmune response, apart from these obvious reasons, it is a mystery to medical doctors and researchers who diagnose and study diseases of autoimmunity.

Bodily Metabolism Depends on Thyroid Hormones

Since both the muscles and nerves are highly dependent upon a normal metabolism to operate correctly, they can become negatively hindered and possibly damaged by thyroid hormone imbalances that are severe or when treatment is delayed for them.

My belief after corresponding with literally 100s of fellow-thyroid patients since the year 2003 is that some patients experience problems with neuropathy and/or myopathy, even after receiving adequate or optimal thyroid treatment and I am in-fact one of them.

The "metabolic aspect" of thyroid disease previously described which causes either a slowed hypothyroid metabolism or a sped-up hyperthyroid metabolism can be a factor that causes development of neuropathy and myopathy as well. This is true even if it is secondarily-caused, rather than being a problem within the thyroid gland itself.

Secondary causes of thyroid dysfunction result from other problems within the body, that affect thyroid hormone production but that still affect bodily metabolism as a result, due to an imbalance in the hormones. If the pituitary gland for example, becomes disrupted due to a tumor that develops within it, this can cause it to either slow-down or speed-up the dispersing of TSH to the thyroid gland.

This is referred to as "central hypothyroidism" and "central hyperthyroidism", meaning there is a problem occurring in the brain-center from which proper thyroid regulation normally originates. In females, tumors on the ovaries can be a secondary cause of an overactive thyroid gland as well.

Small tumors within the thyroid gland itself, called "hot nodules" which would actually be a "primary cause" of hyperthyroidism but that can occur without thyroid autoimmunity being present, can also develop. A long-term, uncorrected abnormal increase or decrease in metabolism due to thyroid hormone imbalances can become detrimental to the body.

Symptoms of Thyroid Hormone Disorders

When <u>hypothyroidism</u> occurs due to any cause, the resulting symptoms can include the following.

• Muscle and joint aches
• Nerve pain in the extremities

• Feeling cold in warm temperatures

• Dry skin and brittle fingernails

• Hair that has become brittle and breaks off or falls out

• Thinning of the eyebrows and loss of the outer 1/3 portion of them

• Unexplained weight gain with no diet change

• Constipation

• Slowed heart rate and breathing

• Depression

• Physical tiredness/fatigue
• Myxedema (fluid retention-tissue swelling)

• Feeling a fullness or tightness in the throat (goiter)

When <u>hyperthyroidism</u> occurs due to any cause, the resulting symptoms can include the following.

• Muscle and joint aches aches (possible muscle atrophy)
• Nerve pain in the extremities ---

- Rapid heart rate
- Hyperventilation
- Hypertension
- Sweating
- Inability to sleep
- Nervousness and anxiety
- Diarrhea
- Excessive energy followed by fatigue
- Hair loss
- Weight loss
- Osteoporosis (bone loss)
- Myxedema
- Swelling of the thyroid gland (goiter)

In many cases the "myxedema" symptom, shown in both lists, is directly related to nerve pain in the body due to fluid-retention causing excessive pressure on the nerves. When either of these thyroid hormone imbalances has been diagnosed, treatment for them will begin. In the chapter that follows, diagnoses methods and treatments will be discussed.

CHAPTER TWO

Treatments for Hypothyroid and Hyperthyroid Hormone Imbalances

For both hypothyroid and hyperthyroid disorders, blood lab testing is often the type of diagnostic method that first detects them. A panel is often ordered when symptoms indicate a thyroid hormone imbalance is present and it will often consist of the T4, T3 and TSH levels.

If additional labs are ordered, these will usually be imaging tests, such as radioactive iodine uptake scans, thyroid ultrasound, MRI, CAT scans and occasionally, a fine-needle tissue biopsy is extracted from the thyroid gland for analysis.

The Sensitivity of TSH Blood Testing

If a thyroid condition is not suspected and a patient is simply having a battery of tests ordered for a routine medical evaluation, the only test that might be included to evaluate thyroid function will be the TSH. This test is often the most sensitive for detecting a lowering or increasing T4 and/or T3 level. The reason for this being, that TSH is increased to abnormally high levels, to maintain proper thyroid hormone levels when they are decreased even slightly, due to a diseased thyroid gland or due to a secondary cause resulting in hypothyroidism.

If the gland has begun to produce too-much thyroid hormone due to primary or secondary hyperthyroidism the opposite will occur.

The TSH will begin to drop to below-normal levels, even early into the thyroid over-activity. During this process, the pituitary gland may be able to correct the T4 and T3 for a period of time but it struggles to do so and eventually the thyroid hormones also become imbalanced, as the TSH fails to maintain them at normal values.

Many patients' thyroid disorders first manifest with an abnormal TSH and the T4 and T3 will remain temporarily-normal at this juncture. This is referred-to as "subclinical thyroid disorder" and for many patients; their condition will stay at a subclinical stage for months or even years.

If a patient experiences symptoms of either overactive or underactive thyroid glands, even when only the TSH is abnormal, some doctors will begin treatment at this stage. If symptoms are not present with an abnormal TSH level, a doctor might instead retest the patients' blood level of TSH, every few months to see if the disorder is progressing to an overt level (full blown).

When Do Doctors Start Treatment for Thyroid Disorders?

Different thyroid-specializing doctors use a different standard for determining when to treat developing hypothyroid and hyperthyroid disorders. Some doctors will treat hypothyroid patients whose TSH is elevated but whose T4 and T3 levels are normal, as long as TSH reaches a level of at-least "10.0" or higher (the highest normal value at labs, currently averages about "5.0").

Some doctors will also treat hypothyroid patients if both the TSH is elevated and the T4 or T3 are below normal on blood test results. Yet other doctors factor-in the presence or absence of symptoms, as previously mentioned.

The same type logic is used by some doctors in regard to hyperthyroid conditions as well but in this case, the TSH lowest normal value averages approximately "0.3" at testing labs, currently. If a hyperthyroid patient has indications of an overactive metabolism (symptoms), with a below-normal TSH but their T4 and T3 remain within normal values, the doctor may opt to start them on treatment as well and most doctors will certainly do-so if both TSH is abnormally low and the T4 and/or T3 are abnormally high.

Types of Thyroid Disease Treatments

Hypothyroidism treatment is relatively simple compared to treatments for hyperthyroidism and consists of simply supplementing the hypothyroid patient with a daily dose of T4 or combination T4 and T3 hormone replacement medication.

The prescribed dose will correct the low thyroid hormone levels over time but this might take a process of several months, with the dose starting at a minimal level and being titrated upward (adjusted by gradual increases), until the patients' TSH, T4 and T3 levels return to adequate or optimal normal values. This is determined via repeat blood testing, every few weeks or months.

Hyperthyroidism treatments are slightly more complicated and varied, depending on the cause of the overactive thyroid gland and the severity of it. In some cases, a patient will only require the prescribing of an "anti-thyroid drug", which slows the production of thyroid hormones, returning thyroid function to a normal level.

Other patients might need a beta-blocker medication prescribed, which will correct hypertension and tachycardia (rapid heart rate) if these are present and if an anti-thyroid drug alone does not correct them. A combination of both type drugs can in some cases, correct the hyperthyroidism symptoms more adequately.

Some hyperthyroid patients need corrective surgeries, to move part or all of their thyroid glands (partial or total thyroidectomy) or they will be referred for radioactive iodine ablation of the gland. This latter mentioned procedure, abbreviated "RAI" is performed by a qualified doctor who administers a dose of radioactive iodine to a patient, which is immediately absorbed by the gland and causes destruction of all tissues within it, so that it is basically dissolved/removed from the body within several weeks following the treatment.

Many doctors are now seeing more value in surgical removal because this often assures that the diseased thyroid tissue is fully removed. Thyroidectomy also becomes necessary in cases of thyroid cancer or when hot nodules are present but in the case of non-malignant nodules, only partial removal may become necessary.

Once thyroid removal of either type has been completed, the patient will require thyroid hormone replacement therapy, similar to that of hypothyroid patients, due to their thyroid glands not being fully present or not present at all, to supply thyroid hormone for proper bodily metabolism.

Is Prescribed Thyroid Hormone Always Adequate?

While these treatments correct thyroid hormone imbalances, some patients may still go on to see progression of neuropathy or myopathy symptoms. As stated earlier, my belief is that the "autoimmune" aspect of thyroid diseases may be responsible for this or it is also possible that supplemented thyroid hormones do not nourish the body and its metabolism as well as do naturally-occurring thyroid hormones.

This second possibility is certainly a theory at this point however, even the pharmaceutical companies who manufacture synthetic and natural brands of prescribed thyroid hormones, claim that certain competing brands do not as adequately resolve the complications of hypothyroid conditions.

Inadequacies in some manufactured hormones have actually resulted in the FDA requiring recalls of certain types, after dosage-inconsistency were found in them (pharmacies required to take the product off-sale). Even the major brand manufacturers have been affected by these recalls in past years.

CHAPTER THREE

Why Thyroid Treatments may not Resolve Neuropathy and Myopathy Symptoms

There are a number of reason why thyroid disease treatments might not fully resolve cases of peripheral neuropathy or thyroid myopathy. As mentioned in the previous chapter, one reason could be that thyroid hormones coming into the body from the outside (prescribed), rather than from the thyroid gland, naturally, may be less adequate.

As also previously mentioned, thyroid hormone replacement is not just required by hypothyroid patients but also by hyperthyroid patients who have had thyroidectomies or radioactive iodine ablations performed on them.

Undertreated Hypothyroid Patients

Some doctors, who are less-qualified to administer thyroid hormone replacement therapy, may also have a tendency to under-treat some patients. This can be due to the concern some doctors have for inducing thyrotoxicity (over-treatment causing hyperthyroidism) and as a result, they are reluctant to optimize treatment for patients to prevent the risk of inducing hyperthyroid symptoms. Under-treated patients carry the risk of complications from what amounts to being kept in a subclinical hypothyroid state by their doctors, including those affecting nerves and muscles.

Once Damage has been Done

I also believe that it's entirely possible that once nerve or muscle damage has occurred in thyroid patients, whether from hyperthyroid or hypothyroid conditions, the treatments they receive may not stop progression of further damage or the preceding damage is not fully reversible.

Medical sources that inform the public about "Thyroid Myopathy", state that the disease can be progressive, similar to types of muscular dystrophy and it becomes a disease entity of itself. Once this occurs, treatments are designed to address symptoms and to comfort patients as much as possible, rather than to reverse the disease process, if it has been established that it is irreversible.

Sensory, Autonomic and Motor Nerves

This same applies to some cases of peripheral neuropathy (PN), which once damaging the nerves, continues to cause sensory symptoms, such as burning, tingling and stabbing pains to the extremities via the "sensory nerves" and that can progress to the trunk of the body and to the nerves that regulate involuntary organ functions as well (autonomic neuropathy).

If the "motor nerves" are also affected by a case of PN (those that affect muscle strength and movement), this may in some cases be placed into the category of a neuromuscular disease.

This is not common and is more likely to occur in thyroid patients with other autoimmune diseases (i.e. Lupus, Rheumatoid Arthritis, Celiac disease and Sjogren 's syndrome) and in those with co-morbid diabetes than in those with thyroid disease only.

In my personal case however, I have had other autoimmune diseases and diabetes ruled-out repeatedly but I continue to experience neuropathy and myopathy symptoms, even after more than eight years of hypothyroid treatment, that has been optimized best-possible.

Research Regarding Neuropathy and Myopathy in Treated Thyroid Patients

Following are quotes from the U.S. National Institutes of Health (PubMed), regarding unresolved neuropathy and myopathy in treated hypothyroid patients, from five different research studies.

1.Pain and small-fiber neuropathy in patients with hypothyroidism (U.S. National Library of Medicine - PubMed) ---

"Conclusions: Some patients treated for hypothyroidism have symptoms and findings compatible with small-fiber neuropathy or "hyper phenomena" indicating central sensitization. ...of Eighteen patients...Eight were classified as having large fiber neuropathy..."

2.Hypothyroidism and polyneuropathy. (U.S. National Library of Medicine - PubMed) ---

"Using standard electrophysiological criteria, a definite diagnosis of polyneuropathy was made in 28 cases (72%). The commonest sites of abnormal nerve conduction were the sensory nerves, especially the sural nerve."

3.Hypothyroid neuropathy and myopathy: clinical and electrodiagnostic longitudinal findings. (U.S. National Library of Medicine - PubMed) ---

"This case shows that thyroid hormone replacement eliminates the neuropathic manifestations of severe hypothyroidism. In contrast, the myopathic features, such as weakness and muscle wasting, may persist despite maintenance of the euthyroid state."

4.Neuromuscular status of thyroid diseases: a prospective clinical and electrodiagnostic study. (U.S. National Library of Medicine - PubMed) ---

Among the thyroid patients, 17 (42.5%) patients were diagnosed with mononeuropathy and polyneuropathy. Entrapment neuropathy was observed in 30% and diffuse neuropathy in 10% of the patients.Myopathy findings were observed in 2 patients.

5.Aspects of peripheral nerve involvement in patients with treated hypothyroidism. (U.S. National Library of Medicine - PubMed) ---

"RESULTS: Sixty-three per cent of the patients with 'pure' hypothyroidism had abnormalities on NCS, 25% had reduced IENF density and 31% had abnormalities on QST. Four patients (25%) met criteria for small fibre polyneuropathy, the other (75%) were classified as having mixed fiber polyneuropathy.

I believe this research makes the point very clear, that not all thyroid patients see recovery from neuropathy or myopathy symptoms, following proper treatment.

Co-morbid Nutritional Deficiencies

A final reason for treated thyroid patients continuing to experience neuropathy and/or myopathy symptoms or actually developing them in spite of being treated, that I will also mention, are "nutritional deficiencies" occurring co-morbid to thyroid disease.

All nutrients, which include vitamins, minerals and electrolytes, have potential to negatively affect nerve and/or muscle function when they become imbalanced and this can be true whether they become deficient or abnormally elevated in the body.

Common deficiencies that are found in thyroid patients include vitamins B12 and D and the mineral-electrolyte deficiencies potassium and magnesium. Others can potentially occur as well however, including deficiencies in other B-vitamins, as well as vitamin E and other types of essential nutrients.

When myopathy and/or neuropathy are occurring in spite of adequate thyroid treatment, a full nutritional blood panel should be ordered. All nutritional deficiencies are treatable and corrective supplementation of nutrients can correct problems in the nerves and muscles that are dependent upon normal levels of them.

Hyperthyroid patients are at risk for developing nutritional deficiencies, due to their sped-up digestion, which causes food to pass through them very quickly. Most patients experience ongoing diarrhea and this can result in malabsorption of essential nutrients over time. Once their hyperthyroidism is corrected, they may still need low nutrients replaced via proper supplementation, as approved by their doctors.

My Own Diagnosis of Thyroid Disease and Deficient Nutrients

My case of Hashimoto's thyroiditis, diagnosed in year-2003 has not been passed down to me from previous generations. Neither my parents, grandparents nor even my great grandparents were known to have autoimmune thyroid disease of any kind. Some medical research, as stated by the AACE (American Association of Endocrinologist), states that thyroid autoimmunity is inherited in approximately 50% of cases that are diagnosed. In my case it is not inherited and my belief is that EBV (the "Epstein - Barr virus" -- that causes mononucleosis) is very possibly a direct cause of my autoimmune hypothyroidism.

The correlations to contracting the virus in my childhood and to my ongoing immune system problems, from that point forward, are simply too striking to be coincidental.

When I was approximately age-10, I became very ill with mononucleosis and I was out of school with the virus for over 6 weeks. My two brothers and my sister never manifested any symptoms of mono, in spite of being in close contact with me during my bout with the illness. Once the viral illnesses had run its course, the glands in my neck returned to normal size, my fever resolved and my fatigue improved. I returned to school and normal activities but my body continued to manifest problems that I now know were related to dysfunction of my immune system. I developed childhood asthma and I experienced colds and viruses, more frequently than did my siblings. I remember on one occasion, my family contracted a respiratory virus and upon all of us our seeing a doctor on the same day, he informed my parents that my case was the most severe.

I mention this regarding EBV, due to the fact that many medical research studies have been published, linking EBV to the development of neurological conditions. This gives me yet one other possibility of a cause for both my thyroid autoimmunity and my co-morbid neuropathy symptoms.

My belief is that autoimmune thyroid diseases are among the common post-viral effects of EBV. I noticed sometime ago, that an Oklahoma-based medical research group, was attempting to patent a vaccination for EBV.

In their statements included on their patent application, they cite the fact that the virus has been implemented as a cause of many different autoimmune diseases. My feeling is that the immune system is adamant about eradicating the body of this virus. When it cannot do-so completely, it may begin to attack major organs or hormone glands that contain the virus, including a person's thyroid gland. This is a theory at this point but one I feel has real merit in light of medical research studies.

My Treatment since Year 2003

In my case as a hypothyroid patient, treated since 2003, with ongoing nerve and muscle symptoms, I was found to be deficient in vitamins D and E and I was found to have insufficient levels of B12 as well (low-normal).

My blood electrolyte level of potassium was found to be slightly below normal and my phosphate became slightly elevated, however, the phosphate normalized with replacing the low vitamin levels, while the potassium required supplementation and diet changes to correct.

Some thyroid patients can benefit from a good daily multivitamin and they can certainly benefit from modifying their diets to include more fruits, vegetables, nuts and grains versus simple carbohydrates which come in the form of junk foods. Regular exercise helps nutrients and hormones to circulate better in the body and helps the body to rid itself of toxins and extra fat that can block some of the positive effects of nutrients.

CHAPTER FOUR

Considering all Treatment Options for Thyroid Neuropathy and Myopathy

Neuropathy and myopathy in thyroid disease patients can be improved in most cases to varied degrees as previously discussed. For some patients, these problems may completely resolve over time, while others may still experience them.

The first consideration in resolving these symptoms best-possible is to make sure thyroid hormone therapies are optimized, best possible. For some thyroid doctors, this means getting the TSH level suppressed into the low-normal or even the lowest-normal value and getting the T4 and T3 levels raised to above mid-range and possibly up to highest-normal values. Needs are varied among different patients and this is why it is important that a qualified doctor is sought for treatment and one who considers each patients' symptoms as well, rather than basing treatment on blood lab values alone.

Getting tested for possible nutritional deficiencies can also be very important as previously mentioned, especially if thyroid hormone correction does not adequately relieve muscle and nerve related symptoms.

Drugs that Treat Nerve and/or Muscle Pain

There are many types of medications, including both the prescribed types and those that can be purchased over-the-counter to help regulate pain involving nerves/muscles.

There are three classes of drugs that are specifically directed at relieving pain in-general, which include the following types and brands.

• **Over-The-Counter Drugs:**

• Acetaminophen

• Aspirin

• ibuprofen

• Naproxen

• **Antidepressants:**

• Tricyclic Antidepressants (TCA's) – (i.e. Types: Amitriptyline and Nortriptiline)

• Selective Serotonin Reuptake Inhibitors (SSRI) – (i.e. Brands: Paxil, Prozac, Zoloft)

• **Anticonvulsants:**

• Gabapentin

• Carbamazepine

• Felbamate

• Valproic Acid ---

• Clonazepam

• Phenytoin

In severe cases of pain, that fails to improve with medication, patients may be referred for "nerve block treatments", which consist of a series of injections into the areas of pain, using a substance such as alcohol or phenol (carbolic acid) to interrupt pain signals. The injections are given at regular intervals, to help with ongoing, severe pain.

Nerve Entrapment Therapies

When pain is referred from a nerve that is being pinched (nerve entrapment), treatments will be directed at relieving the pressure on the affected nerves. Some nerve entrapments cause significant pain, such as those affecting the "sciatic nerve" (a large nerve that runs from the back, into the legs and feet), the "median nerve" (affecting the wrists and hands) and the posterior tibial nerve (affecting the feet and toes).

Treatments may include surgical procedures, massage and chiropractic therapies, temperature applications (ice packs or heating pads) and isolation, meaning a period of restricted or non-movement of limbs or other body-parts that contain entrapped nerves (movement may be encouraged if muscles are primarily affected). In some cases, nerve-stimulation devices are used in attempt to stimulate proper impulses from nerves that have been affected by long-term entrapment.

It is important to see a qualified medical doctor for the evaluation and treatment of thyroid disorders and for referral to treatments for co-morbid problems affecting the nerves and/or muscles, when thyroid treatment alone does not resolve them. I offer my most sincere "best wishes" to the readers of this book, who are seeking treatment-solutions for their thyroid-related myopathies and neuropathies.

(END) --*See the bonus chapter following, for a little humor (very little).*

CHAPTER FIVE

Eight Thyroid Disease Knock-Knock Jokes: (Laughing at the Expense of the Metabolic Butterfly)

Some readers might think "What! – A thyroid disease joke chapter – you've got to be kidding!" and I would respond by saying "Yes, I am kidding and that's the purpose of this chapter!" We're doing something that comedy often does, by taking a serious subject and finding a way to laugh about it. Why not?!

As thyroid patients who go through the ups and downs of our diseases, why shouldn't we find a way to derive some humor from it? I believe by doing so, that we can actually find better coping as we may sometimes struggle with the fact that we're living with a lifelong disease that will require ongoing treatment for most of us, as we live-out our lives in this world.

What better way is there, to take some of the seriousness out of the fear we sometimes experience when we're having a flare of symptoms or we're experiencing some emotional phases with our diseases, than to find ways to laugh about it?

It is my sincere hope that fellow-patients or anyone who enjoys a good laugh will do-so, while reading this added bonus-chapter. As a patient with autoimmune thyroiditis that is causing me lifelong hypothyroidism and co morbid health problems, plus a need for daily treatments for it, I feel that laughter truly is a good medicine.

149

It can help me to cope better, when I'm feeling a bit down due to my disease and its symptoms. I hope this proves to be the case for those who read this chapter as well!

While some of these knock-knock jokes are a bit on the corny side (some smack in the middle of it), I think they will still get you to smile a little and hopefully some of them will get a few genuine giggles out of you. So, with the boring chapter-introduction out of the way, let's get to the comedy.

Knock-knock

Who's there?

I Goiter

I goiter who?

I goiter go to the doctor, cause my neck feels swollen.

Knock-knock

Who's there?

R.U. Goins

R.U. Goins who?

R.U. Goins to the doctor, cause your mood seems like it's hypothyroid.

150

Knock-knock

Who's there?

I.M. Crabbie

I.M. Crabbie who?

I.M. crabbie because I forgot to take my thyroid pill this morning.

_____

Knock-knock

Who's there?

B.A. Angel

B.A. Angel who?

B.A. angel and order me a double cheeseburger, my hypothyroidism is making me hungry.

_____

Knock-knock

Who's there?

B4 U

B4 U Who?

B4 U call me a zombie, remember that I might be having brain fog.

Knock-knock

Who's there?

I.R. Moody

I.R. Moody who?

I.R. Moody today, so don't push your luck by pushing my buttons.

Knock-knock

Who's there?

I.B. Shedding

I.B. Shedding who?

I.B. Shedding hair, so don't mistake my pillow for a raccoon in the bed.

Knock-knock

Who's there?

152

M.I. Goen

M.I. Goen who?

M.I. goen to the doctor soon, cause my thyroid hormone pills don't seem to be working?

_____

(END - Section Four)

SECTION FIVE

The Depression of Hypothyroidism

Mood Problems from Untreated or Undertreated Thyroid

To all of my fellow hypothyroid patients, who struggle with low mood issues as I have. It is my prayer for you, to find peace of mind and victory over your feelings of chronic depression. It is also my hope to inspire you toward successful coping and treatment through the words I offer within the pages of this book.

TABLE OF CONTENTS:

INTRODUCTION:

If I were to personally name the symptom I believe to be the most life-altering and the one that causes the most anguish resulting from the disease of hypothyroidism, I would have to say that for me and likely for many other hypothyroid patients, "depression" would be that symptom. Certainly anxiety can also be present in hypothyroid patients and medical research studies have revealed this fact clearly.

While anxiety commonly occurs together to varying degrees with depression, true clinical depression is often the emotional disorder that can more-often lead one to severe states of anguish, hopelessness and despair.

It is in fact a major cause of suicide throughout the world according to medical statistics and this is just as true of hypothyroid patients who can experience ongoing struggles with this sometimes debilitating emotional issue as I have with my own autoimmune hypothyroidism (Hashimoto's thyroiditis).

Within the chapters that follow, I wish to address this emotional symptom of an underactive thyroid gland, including descriptions of how it manifests and how hypothyroid patients can deal with it and have it treated successfully to regain an improved quality of life.

I will also include medical research study quotes, found on the U.S. National Institutes of Health medical research information website (PubMed), which allows reprints for public education purposes.

It is my sincere hope that this information proves to be helpful to hypothyroid patients seeking information regarding stubborn symptoms of depression that do not resolve for them adequately in spite of being treated for their hypothyroidism.

(NOTE: Some lifestyle practices information regarding goitrogen foods, supplements and diet are repeated from "SECTION TWO" which was on the subject of "Thyroid Cancer".)

-*Jim Lowrance*

CHAPTER ONE

How Does Depression Manifest in Hypothyroid Patients?

Symptoms of low mood actually manifest and are experienced by hypothyroid patients, the same as they are by those who suffer clinical depression for any other reasons that are medical or due to life circumstances. A major aspect of depression is simply the fact that it extracts the motivation to do positive things from the individual affected by it but it may in some cases also inspire a person toward negative behaviors and actions (i.e. violence, rejection of love and suicide).

In the case of it hindering positive traits in a person, this would include things such as accomplishing tasks at work or school, being creative with artistic pursuits, such as writing, painting or sculpting and being unable to enjoy things that were formerly indulged-in, such as family events, hobbies and even sexual gratification with one's spouse.

In many cases, a person with clinical depression will experience a profound sadness that causes them to have frequent crying spells or to feel emotionally negative even over mildly adverse events that might arise or transpire in their lives.

Other depression sufferers will report that they actually feel emotionally numb, so that neither feelings of love or sadness are apparent to them but they rather feel void of almost all emotion that they would normally experience in response to daily life events both negative and positive.

When clinical depression is severe, it can unfortunately cause very severe reactions in those experiencing it when adverse life-events do occur, such as the loss of a loved one or a long-held position with an employer or following a financial crises. In these cases, depressed people may begin to contemplate suicide and others may actually resort to the very act of it. This is why it is so important for one who feels they are slipping into a severe state of depression, to seek help immediately and for those who may observe behaviors in a loved one with depression, to seek help for them and to do-so even with possible protest by them toward receiving any help.

Rejecting help is often a denial aspect also experienced by sufferers of depression, who can find it very difficult to accept the fact that they are experiencing emotional problems in need of medical and/or psychiatric attention. It can often help in such cases, to reassure the person, that their need for help is nothing to be ashamed-of or embarrassed about because they are experiencing a medical problem that is of no fault of their own and that they are far from being alone with this very common emotional disorder (affecting 1 in every 5 people by some estimates). It can also be important for them to understand that getting help for their mood disorder, is not only for their sake but also for the sake of their loved ones who are concerned for their well being.

Some additional manifestations of depression which can also be crossover symptom similarities between low mood and unresolved hypothyroid symptoms from untreated or under-treated hypothyroidism, can include the following:

• Fatigue and body weakness ---

• The need to sleep more than normal

• Mild to moderate general body pain

• Stress headaches & difficulty concentrating

• Low libido (sex drive)

Obviously, the recommended treatments for depression in-general, would include psychotropic medications and psychiatric therapies (i.e. antidepressants and Cognitive Behavioral Therapy) and for some people one treatment or the other may be effective, while some benefit more from a combination of both. With the fact that depression can actually be caused directly by hypothyroidism and is often mistaken for mood disorder, without an underlying medical cause and with the fact that "inadequately treated hypothyroidism" can cause depression and other symptoms of low metabolism to remain unresolved, I will address the importance of optimal "thyroid hormone replacement therapy", within the chapters that follow.

I would like to add some important statements in closing this first chapter, by saying that many hypothyroid patients are treated very adequately by their doctors or what we might also call "optimally" but they still need the added help of psychotropic drugs or psychiatric therapies to see resolution for clinical depression. The need for such added treatments can be necessary while waiting for hypothyroid treatment to be fully realized by a patient (awaiting the full effect which can take several months) or once treatment is confirmed to be optimal via blood retests of thyroid hormone therapy levels and symptom-monitoring.

These additional treatments may still be found to be necessary for unresolved depression (sometimes trial and error are required to find what works best for individual patients).

Since this book is about depression associated with hypothyroidism, I will mainly concentrate the content on that aspect of treating clinical depression.

CHAPTER TWO

My Hypothyroid Depression Story

My own case of hypothyroidism is caused by a common form of autoimmune thyroiditis called "chronic lymphocytic thyroiditis" (Hashimoto's disease). It is an immune system caused disease in which specially created cells designed to destroy intruders in the body, such as germs, bacteria and allergy causing cells, are attacked and rendered incapable of performing the dirty tasks of making us sick.

For some reason however, these immune cells begin to be created to attack good tissues and organs in our bodies, that pose no threat to us at all, in fact that instead, actually help our bodies to operate as a healthy system. The thyroid gland can be one of the organs/glands that begins to be on the receiving-end of this autoimmune attack and medical research has yet to understand fully, as to why this happens.

I have a theory as a layperson on the subject, that comes from my own ongoing search (since year 2003) regarding autoimmune diseases and in-particular, those affecting the thyroid gland and I have come to the non-professional opinion, that attacks of autoimmunity, that causes diseases such as thyroid disorders, autoimmune forms of arthritis, multi-system connective tissue diseases like lupus and many others, are due to there actually being something within human tissues that is never fully eradicated from the body by the immune system.

Different types of diseases that are contracted during childhood for example, such as the Epstein-Barr Virus ("EBV" -- the cause of mononucleosis) and chicken pox, actually remain within the body for long periods of time or life-long, although they become dormant (present but not actively causing the same initial illness).

Some medical information sources actually state that EBV is present in up to 95% of the general population, regardless of whether only a small percent of them actually suffered from mono symptoms when they initially contracted the disease. This means they become carriers able to infect others with the virus regardless of whether or not they actually became ill or not. I feel that these viruses that remain inside the bodies of relatively healthy individuals, can eventually cause the immune system, which is designed to protect us from them, to go into overdrive or to become confused at some point and to begin attacking normal tissues within the body that continue to hold these virus cells.

With the inability of the immune system to fully eradicate these invaders, it then begins to design immune cells to attack the very tissues they live in. While this is an unproven theory at this point, there have been many studies conducted by medical groups, many of which can be seen on sources such as PubMed (U.S. National Institutes of Health Website), that have shown a well-established association of childhood viruses to the development of autoimmune diseases. In recent years, EBV was found to be highly associated with the development of Multiple Sclerosis in controlled research studies as well.

Before my ever finding this information through my own search/research, I was already wondering if my severe case of mononucleosis as a child, resulted in significant immune function changes, that affected me later in life and caused me to develop hypothyroidism in year-2003 at age 40. I actually mention this in other books I have authored and one reader who added a review under one of them stated that my mention of EBV being connected to thyroid disease was somewhat far-fetched. I was a bit taken-back by that statement, especially with the fact that some of the research I refer to above, specifically associates (strongly connects) EBV to the development of autoimmune thyroid disease specifically.

Here is a research quote from PubMed (this and other reprints I will cite in this book, are allowed for educational purposes):

"Epstein-Barr virus serology in patients with autoimmune thyroiditis.

Source: Institute of Endocrinology, Prague, Czech Republic.

Abstract

Elevated titers of antibodies against different antigens of Epstein-Barr virus (EBV) are found in some immunodeficient states, malignancies or in autoimmune disorders. We examined EBV serology in the group of 22 patients with autoimmune thyroiditis as compared with the group of 35 healthy volunteers. ---

Titers of antibodies against viral capsid antigen (IgG-VCA) were more often found in the group of patients than in the control group (p = 0.000 35 for younger than 40 years and p = 0.00115 for older than 40 years) and the positivity of antibodies against early antigen (IgG-EA-D/DR) was also significantly more often found in the group of patients (p = 0.0031 and p = 0.0019 respectively) than in the control group."

While the above quoted abstract of the research study I have given, does not state specifically that EBV caused thyroid autoimmunity in the participants studied, the finding is significant and obviously points to the virus as being a suspected, direct cause of autoimmune thyroid disease. It is also true that some people develop a sub-acute form of thyroiditis (sudden, severe but temporary) caused by upper respiratory viral infections and this too, would suggest that viral illnesses do indeed play a role in the later development of autoimmune thyroid disorders. Yet other medical studies state that emotional disorders can result not only from thyroid hormone imbalances but also from the actual thyroid autoimmunity.

Following is another PubMed quote which points out the role of thyroid autoimmunity in mood disorders, including both the anxiety and depression types:

"Background:

Autoimmune thyroid disease may be linked to depression and anxiety. Autoimmune disease and depression are not uncommon: ---

---

the prevalence of autoimmune thyroid disease in the community ranged from 4 to 25% and lifetime prevalence of Major Depressive Disorder ranged from 6 to 17%. Thus the association may have a great relevance in terms of public health and prevention.

Conclusions

The study seems to suggest that individuals in the community with thyroid autoimmunity may be at high risk for mood and anxiety disorders. The psychiatric disorders and the autoimmune reaction seem to be rooted in a same (and not easy correctable) aberrancy in the immuno-endocrine system. Should our results be confirmed, the findings may be of great interest for future preventive and case finding projects."

(From the research Abstract titled: "The link between thyroid autoimmunity (antithyroid peroxidase autoantibodies) with anxiety and mood disorders in the community: a field of interest for public health in the future")

In referring back to my earlier mention of contracting mono from EBV, I was approximately age-10 when this occurred and my siblings (2 brothers and 1 sister) were almost certainly also infected but none of them developed mono as I did. My case was severe and caused me to be taken out of school for approximately six weeks as I recovered from the illness. Afterward, I began to experience colds and other viruses on a more severe level than did other members of my family and I developed asthma, digestive problems and a case of anemia at one point as well.

I also developed a heart murmur in my teens which I now believe to have been the beginnings of a condition called Mitral Valve Prolapse ("MVP" - common in the general population), which medical studies have found to be more common in people with thyroid autoimmunity than in the general population and that some medical sources believe to possibly be an autoimmune condition itself.

Following is a research quote from PubMed, indicating this finding:

"Mitral valve prolapse in autoimmune thyroid disease: an index of systemic autoimmunity?

Source: Department of Medical Therapeutics, Alexandra Hospital, Athens University School of Medicine, Greece.

Abstract

A coexistence of mitral valve prolapse (MVP) with autoimmune thyroid disease (AITD) has been described, but there are not sufficient data to explain this association. The aim of the present study was to investigate the prevalence of MVP in patients with AITD and to evaluate whether any correlation between MVP and certain immunological parameters exists. M-mode, two-dimensional Doppler echocardiography was performed in 29 patients with Graves' disease (GD), 35 with Hashimoto's thyroiditis (HT), 20 with nonautoimmune goiter, and 30 normal controls.

Serum samples were examined for antinuclear antibodies (ANA), antibodies against extractable nuclear antigen (ENA), antiphospholipid antibodies (aCL), rheumatoid factor (RF), thyroid autoantibodies(TAAb), immunoglobulins and C3, C4.

Eight of 29 GD patients and 8 of 35 HT patients had MVP, while none of the control group and 2 of 20 of the simple goiter group had MVP (p < 0.05). ANA were detected at low titers in 5 of 8 in MVP(+) GD versus 3 of 21 in MVP(-) GD (p < 0.05). In the HT group the MVP(+) patients had a significantly higher incidence of ANA and ENA, 5 of 8 and 2 of 8 versus 5 of 27 and 0 of 27 of MVP(-) patients, respectively, p < 0.05.

A statistically significant higher incidence of aCL was found in HT MVP(+) patients. (3/8) versus HT MVP(-) 1/27, p < 0.05. RF levels (immunoglobulin A [IgA]) were significantly higher in MVP(+) patients. The association of MVP with nonorgan-specific autoantibodies indicates that MVP may also be an autoimmune disease. It is possible that patients with AITD who also have MVP may be at an increased risk to develop systemic autoimmunity."

Note the statement within the above-quoted study in particular that says: "The association of MVP with nonorgan-specific autoantibodies indicates that MVP may also be an autoimmune disease". My purpose in adding this fact about MVP, is due to its potential to cause or aggravate already existing depression in people suffering from co-morbid diseases or from mood disorders with no other medical causes and because the estimates of people who may actually have the usually benign cardiac condition are incredibly high (some say as high as 20% of the population). This heart murmur, also referred to as a "click murmur" due to the sound it sometimes presents, when a doctor listens for it through a stethoscope, has depression commonly listed as a symptom for it.

Some medical sources believe that the mood aspect of the condition, may be due to imbalances it causes in some patients, within the involuntary nervous system, which is medically referred to as "dysautonomia".

Some treated hypothyroid patients who also suffer from symptoms of MVP, which is actually called Mitral Valve Proplapse Syndrome" or "MVP-Dysautonomia", may find that even optimal treatment of their hypothyroidism, does not resolve all of their low mood problems. With this being the case, despite the fact that medical information sources state that most cases of MVP do not require treatment, other than healthy lifestyle changes, this may require even more diligence by treated hypothyroid patients like myself, to see better resolution for their depression relief needs (more on the subject of health practices will begin in the next chapter).

For MVP patients who do need drug treatments, these will usually be "beta-blocker" class medications (usually prescribed for hypertension and heart palpitations) and possibly supplementation with magnesium (a mineral-electrolyte important to heart function that can become low in MVP patients) , otherwise the healthy lifestyle changes that can help with symptoms of the click-murmur are basically the same as those recommended for hypothyroid patients.

There are aspects of treatments, that can help those suffering from hypothyroidism related depression to see better gains over this often life-altering struggle with emotional symptoms that can linger even when prescribed thyroid hormone therapy is adhered-to faithfully, as prescribed by a qualified physician.

To finish my reference to my own case in this regard, I saw fairly early relief of both anxiety and depression with my own thyroid hormone therapy however, over the years, I have fluctuated back into depressed and anxious moods for weeks and months at a time. My feelings are that this may indeed have to do with changes in levels of the thyroid antibodies that caused my disease (most likely increases in them) and possibly from changes in thyroid hormone levels as well.

This is why I follow the treatment options I describe in the chapters following, best-possible to prevent emotional symptoms from recurring. I have seen the positive effects these practices can achieve but I have also seen the negative impact that can occur when I fail to practice them (my weaknesses are in regard to proper diet and exercise, while healthy supplements are the easy aspects for me).

CHAPTER THREE

Getting Thyroid Hormone Therapy as Perfected as Possible

There are two partners involved in the treatment of hypothyroidism, being the patient and the doctor. The responsibility of the doctor, is to treat a patient's low thyroid hormones, in order to get them to the best possible level for relieving hypothyroid symptoms, one of which can be chronic, clinical depression. The responsibility of the patient, is to take their prescribed hormone therapy, as directed by their doctor and to report any symptoms changes to him. The patient should also follow the healthiest possible lifestyle practices, which directly impact the effectiveness of their hormone replacement therapy.

Following is another medical research article excerpt from PubMed, that honestly recognizes the inadequacies that can occur with hypothyroid treatment, due to a variety of possible reasons:

"We tell our patients, "It's really quite simple, your thyroid is not working (or has been removed or destroyed by our treatment). The tablet contains the natural hormone that your body cannot make. Don't worry, you'll be fine." For many of our patients, T4 therapy resolves their symptoms and they are fine. For some, however, this therapy remains unsatisfactory, with the persistence of specific symptoms or a failure to regain a normal sense of well-being.

....

More needs to be done to understand why some patients do not feel completely well on what, according to current standards, is adequate thyroid hormone replacement. First, careful cross-sectional and/or case-control epidemiological studies are needed to develop a standardized definition of cases, determine their prevalence, and generate testable hypotheses. Second, efforts should continue to identify molecular measurements that indicate, directly or as surrogate markers, whether tissue levels of thyroid hormone are normal.

Third, additional clinical studies with the following characteristics are needed: 1) The study population should be homogeneous. Although this may prevent generalizing the findings, the current uncertainties necessitate starting in this way. 2) The sample size should be large enough to assure that either positive or negative findings can be accepted with confidence. The principal psychological, physiological, and molecular endpoints should be selected with care, and the analysis should take into account the effects of multiple testing. 3) If practical, a random order, double-blind crossover design should be used. 4) In studies to test T3, sustained release preparations, if available, or divided doses should be used. Consideration needs to be given to the implications of a fixed vs. variable T4/T3 ratio in combination therapy, both in regard to study design and therapeutic effect. 5) TSH should be monitored dynamically and study medications adjusted according to the results, to maintain normal serum TSH concentrations."

(From the study titled: "In Search of the Impossible Dream? Thyroid Hormone Replacement Therapy That Treats All Symptoms in All Hypothyroid Patients")

The preceding quoted study, points out the importance in more research being conducted regarding "T3 thyroid hormone supplementation" and how it can possibly be more beneficial in some patients than is T4 therapy alone (many doctors already prescribe combination T4 and T3 hormone drugs to their hypothyroid patients). It also points out that T3 therapy can possibly be more customized to patients for better results. The problem of course arises from the fact that many doctors simply do not have the time to better-customize their patient's hypothyroid hormone therapies (the "one-size-fits-all" mentality).

This is where patient-input becomes so important (self-advocacy) because doctors often will not suggest a trial of a different type or brand of thyroid hormone, unless their patients specifically request it (simply a fact). In some cases, a trial of T3 added to a patient's treatment, will not relieve their symptoms better, including depression (some medical studies have shown that T3 therapy can add antidepressant benefit for some hypothyroid and non-hypothyroid patients). Some hypothyroid patients may actually feel better taking a T4 only brand of hormone however, it is not possible to know what an outcome will be, unless a carefully monitored trial is given to see what different hormone combinations may do for a patient with stubborn depression.

Another factor that may become a consideration, is the fact that most patients with hypothyroidism are prescribed a T-4 only brand of thyroid hormone medication (e.i. Synthroid, Levothyroxine) and the needed T-3 hormone is converted from it, within the body successfully. In patients with a less common problem called "impaired conversion" however, a T-4 only hormone medication will not supply them with adequate T-3 that is also needed in the body.

If this problem exists, it will be evident by their blood test results that monitor their dose. If a patient's T-4 to T-3 ratio is off too much they may need a thyroid hormone replacement medication that contains both T-4 and T-3 hormones (e.i. Armour Thyroid, Thyrolar) or they may add a T-3 medication (e.i. Cytomel) to a T-4 only brand they are already taking.

There are also people who by taking a T-4/T-3 combination drug, elevate their Free T-3 level too high and have to be switched to a T-4 only medication. This is why it is important for hypothyroid patients to be treated by qualified doctors, who can determine the type of thyroid hormone medication that is best suited for them. The AACE (American College of Clinical Endocrinologists/Thyroid Specialists) and other medical authorities recommend that hypothyroid patient's TSH levels while on thyroid hormone replacement medication, be suppressed down to between "1.0 and 2.0" (A hormone released by the pituitary gland that reflects thyroid function when blood tested).

The TSH level rises, when thyroid hormone decreases and it falls when the thyroid hormone levels increase. If a patient's TSH is not kept below 2.0, they risk continued hypothyroid symptoms such as depression and if it is brought significantly below 1.0, they risk development of hyperthyroid symptoms (dose-induced thyrotoxicity). Some Endocrinologists actually keep some patient's TSH levels between, "0.3 to 1.0" (lowest normal), as long as this does not cause their T4 and/or T3 level to rise above normal (between mid-range and highest-normal is where they usually like to see these).

Tips for Taking Thyroid Hormone Medication for Best Results

People taking thyroid hormone replacement medication for hypothyroidism need to follow a set routine for taking their medication. Hormone therapy can have a delicate balance; even small variations in the levels created in the body from taking a hormone medication can greatly affect how well a patient feels.

The steps below help to insure the best results from thyroid hormone replacement therapy.

Take your thyroid hormone medication on an empty stomach, with plenty of water. Many patients find it easier to take their thyroid medication on an empty stomach by doing so first thing in the morning before having breakfast. Once the medication has been taken, it is recommended that a patient wait at least 30 minutes before eating, to allow the medication time to be absorbed in the digestive tract. Taking the medication with a full glass of water also helps digestion and absorption of the medication.

Take your thyroid hormone medication at the same time each day. When you take your thyroid medication at the same time each day, this helps your hormone levels remain more stable than if you take it at different times each day. Most thyroid medications have a long half-life of several days. However, even very small changes in the rhythm of your dosage can affect the way you feel. According to the manufacturers of thyroid medications, the hormone will peak in the body at a certain time after ingesting it and then remain stable for a period of time and afterward have a slightly lowered effect.

A patient will want to see the peak and stable effects during the day and the lowered effect toward the end of the day, as time for rest and sleep arrives after a day of activities.

If you take vitamins or supplements containing iron or calcium, be sure to take them six hours apart from your thyroid medication dose. These two supplements can have a negative effect on thyroid hormone medication, by preventing it from fully absorbing in the body as briefly described in a previous heading. To prevent malabsorption, it is recommended that you take these supplements at least six hours apart from your thyroid medication each day (some sources suggest eight hours as a precaution). Some patients take their thyroid medication in the morning on an empty stomach and will take their supplements containing iron and/or calcium after lunch, six hours later, to prevent this problem.

When you have blood retests of your thyroid hormone levels, take your medication at the same time, to correlate with each blood draw. Some patients on the day of a blood draw (to retest their thyroid hormone levels) will skip their thyroid medication dose until after their blood is drawn. Other patients will take their thyroid medication dose before the blood draw but will make sure the blood is drawn at the same time for each retest, to make sure levels are consistent in correlation with it. It really is not that important which method you use, as long as you do so consistently for each blood draw to retest your thyroid hormone levels while being treated for hypothyroidism.

Never adjust your own thyroid medication dose. There can be times when symptoms may manifest themselves despite the fact that you are taking your thyroid medication properly. This might make some patients believe that a slight increase in their dose that day would help relieve these symptoms, and consequently they are tempted to take it upon themselves to increase their dose. This is never a good idea, without the consent and supervision of your doctor; even small adjustments in your dose can alter your hormone levels for days at a time. If a patient seems to be experiencing symptoms of low thyroid hormone or those of an overactive thyroid (too much hormone), they should report these to their doctor for instructions on adjusting their medication or in making an office visit for further evaluation of their treatment.

CHAPTER FOUR

Diet, Supplements and Exercise

Supplementing with Selenium

One nutrient that has also been covered in medical research studies, regarding supplements that can decrease thyroid disease activity, is "selenium", which is both a mineral and an electrolyte that is essential in the body. According to these research studies, the mineral actually "modifies" levels of the antibodies that cause thyroid diseases as discussed earlier. The two major thyroid antibodies, also called "auto-antibodies", that attack key proteins within the gland, causing diseases such as Hashimoto's thyroiditis and Graves' disease, are the "anti-thyroidperoxidase" (immune cells that attack thethyroidperoxidase enzyme/protein – abbreviated "Anti-TPO") and the "anti-thyroglobulin" (immune cells that attack the thyroglobulin enzyme/protein – abbreviated anti-TG).

Selenium, supplemented as a daily regimen, is cited in these studies as having the ability to reduce the TPO antibodies, thereby reducing disease activity in the thyroid gland and the associated inflammation that is also involved.

Research citing selenium as a modifier of thyroid autoimmunity activity:

"In areas with severe selenium deficiency there is a higher incidence of thyroiditis due to a decreased activity of selenium-dependent glutathione peroxidase activity within thyroid cells. ---

Selenium-dependent enzymes also have several modifying effects on the immune system. Therefore, even mild selenium deficiency may contribute to the development and maintenance of autoimmune thyroid diseases.

We performed a blinded, placebo-controlled, prospective study in female patients (n = 70; mean age, 47.5 +/- 0.7 yr) with autoimmune thyroiditis and thyroid peroxidase antibodies (TPOAb) and/or Tgantibodies (TgAb) above 350 IU/ml. The primary end point of the study was the change in TPOAb concentrations. Secondary end points were changes in TgAb, TSH, and free thyroid hormone levels as well as ultrasound pattern of the thyroid and quality of life estimation.

Patients were randomized into 2 age- and antibody (TPOAb)-matched groups; 36 patients received 200 microg (2.53 micromol) sodium selenite/d, orally, for 3 months, and 34 patients received placebo. All patients were substituted with L-T(4) to maintain TSH within the normal range. TPOAb, TgAb, TSH, and free thyroid hormones were determined by commercial assays. The echogenicity of the thyroid was monitored with high resolution ultrasound. The mean TPOAb concentration decreased significantly to 63.6% (P = 0.013) in the selenium group vs. 88% (P = 0.95) in the placebo group.

A subgroup analysis of those patients with TPOAb greater than 1200 IU/ml revealed a mean 40% reduction in the selenium-treated patients compared with a 10% increase in TPOAb in the placebo group.TgAb concentrations were lower in the placebo group at the beginning of the study and significantly further decreased (P = 0.018), but were unchanged in the selenium group.

Nine patients in the selenium-treated group had completely normalized antibody concentrations, in contrast to two patients in the placebo group (by chi(2) test, P = 0.01). Ultrasound of the thyroid showed normalized echogenicity in these patients. The mean TSH, free T(4), and free T(3) levels were unchanged in both groups. We conclude that selenium substitution may improve the inflammatory activity in patients with autoimmune thyroiditis, especially in those with high activity.

Whether this effect is specific for autoimmune thyroiditis or may also be effective in other endocrine autoimmune diseases has yet to be investigated."

Source Link: http://www.ncbi.nlm.nih.gov/pubmed/11932302 (Selenium supplementation in patients with autoimmune thyroiditis decreases thyroid peroxidase antibodies concentrations.")

Exercise a Natural Depression Reliever

Certainly, a recommendation that is always given to thyroid patients by their doctors is to live the healthiest lives possible, to include proper diet and exercise, in addition to getting proper rest and sleep.

The exercise aspect is somewhat obvious and self-explanatory and would include the warning that one should exercise only to tolerance-level and to not overdo when undertaking a regimen, whether of the aerobic or strength and endurance types.

Following is a research quote from a PubMed article regarding the benefits of regular exercise in relieving depression:

"Many studies have examined the efficacy of exercise to reduce symptoms of depression, and the overwhelming majority of these studies have described a positive benefit associated with exercise involvement. For example, 30 community-dwelling moderately depressed men and women were randomly assigned to an exercise intervention group, a social support group, or a wait-list control group.17 The exercise intervention consisted of walking 20 to 40 minutes 3 times per week for 6 weeks. The authors reported that the exercise program alleviated overall symptoms of depression and was more effective than the other 2 groups in reducing somatic symptoms of depression (reduction of 2.4 [walking] vs. 0.9 [social support] and 0.4 [control] on the Beck Depression Inventory [BDI], p < .05). Doyne et al.18 utilized a multiple baseline design to evaluate the effectiveness of interval training in alleviating symptoms of depression. The participants exercised on a cycle ergometer 4 times per week, 30 minutes per session, for 6 weeks. This treatment was compared with an attention-placebo control condition in which subjects listened to audiotapes of "white noise" that they were told was subliminal assertiveness training. Results indicated that the aerobic training program was associated with a clear reduction in depression compared with the control condition, and the improvements in depression were maintained at 3 months post intervention (BDI mean reduction of 14.4 points from baseline, p < .05). ---

In another study, just 30 minutes of treadmill walking for 10 consecutive days was sufficient to produce a clinically relevant and statistically significant reduction in depression (reduction of 6.5 points from baseline on the Hamilton Rating Scale for Depression [HAM-D], $p < .01$).

Research also suggests that the benefits of exercise involvement may be long lasting.20 Depressed adults who took part in a fitness program displayed significantly greater improvements in depression, anxiety, and self-concept than those in a control group after 12 weeks of training (BDI reduction of 5.1 [fitness program] vs. 0.9 [control], $p < .001$). The exercise participants also maintained many of these gains through the 12-month follow-up period."

(From the research article titled: " The Benefits of Exercise for the Clinically Depressed")

The diet aspect of better thyroid health would of course include the recommendation to avoid junk foods (simple carbohydrates -- foods high in saturated fats and high levels of manufactured sugars) and to eat healthy, complex carbohydrates (fruits, vegetables, nuts and grains) however, thyroid patients should avoid certain types of foods that in the long run, can help the thyroid gland to not suffer as severely from autoimmunity that contributes to worsening thyroiditis and hypothyroidism. This would include the avoidance of "goitrogen foods" of which "soy" is a major one and that can be a by-product found in many food-products but is often not recognized unless ingredients are carefully read on food product labels (i.e. soybeans, tofu, soybean oil, soy flour, soy lecithin).

183

Other goitrogen foods include the following:

- cassava
- Pine nuts
- Peanuts
- Millet
- Strawberries
- Pears
- Peaches
- Spinach
- Bamboo shoots
- Sweet Potatoes
- Bok choy
- Broccoli
- Broccolini (Asparations)
- Brussels sprouts
- Cabbage
- Canola
- Cauliflower
- Chinese cabbage
- Choy sum ---

- Collard greens

- Horseradish

- Kai-lan (Chinese broccoli)

- Kale

- Kohlrabi

- Mizuna

- Mustard greens

- Radishes

- Rapeseed (yu choy)

- Rapini

- Rutabagas

- Tatsoi

- Turnips

Some medical sources state that the goitrogen effect of these foods, can be reduced considerably when they are cooked properly (those that require cooking) and when those who have thyroid disease, consume them in moderation (especially those foods that don't require being cooked).

All thyroid patients should also undergo testing of major vitamin levels (i.e. D, B12, E and B6) and other nutrients (i.e. minerals, protein and electrolyte levels).

Deficiencies can be present, without necessarily causing any suggestive symptoms or mood changes may develop as the only symptom of them. Patients, who are diagnosed with hypothyroidism and are being treated for it with hormone replacement therapy, can sometimes have other imbalances that hinder the effectiveness of the treatment. Things such as adrenal hormones being low or low levels of ferritin/iron, Vitamin B-12 etc... (elements needed for strong blood), can cause thyroid hormone treatment, to be less effective in patients with imbalances of these and is why thorough blood testing of all levels may need to be done, to find any problems that prevent the treatment from working as well. Once any deficiencies have been determined, supplementation of the needed nutrients can be highly beneficial in reducing depression symptoms and in helping replacement thyroid hormones to work more optimally within the body.

While I have covered the subjects within these chapters generally, I have give some detail to some aspects. A very important component involved, as mentioned previously, is partnering with your doctor the best possible and to self-advocate, meaning to stand up for yourself respectfully when you feel the need to suggest a change or addition to your treatment that may better improve or alleviate your depression symptoms.

(End - Section Five)

SECTION SIX:

Medically and Spiritually Treating Chronic Thyroid Disease Anxiety

Treatment Experiences and Informed Medical Advice from a Christian Perspective

To all of my fellow thyroid patients, who are seeking peace in the midst of their storms -- may you find your peace restored and your joy recovered as God plants his eternal hope within your heart.

"For our light affliction, which is but for a moment, worketh for us a far more exceeding and eternal weight of glory" (2 Corinthians 4:17 KJV)

TABLE OF CONTENTS:

INTRODUCTION:

While it might seem unusual to see a book title on the subject of offering Christian encouragement to thyroid patients, it really shouldn't be considered unusual at all. Statistics by reputable polling organizations have shown that 75% of the U.S. population claims to be of the Christian faith and some medical estimates have revealed that over 30-million Americans are experiencing thyroid diseases.

General statistics of belief in God are considerably high, with some polling data indicating that 9 out of 10 Americans believe in a supreme being. Some polls that have concentrated on particular groups of people have revealed similar statistics. In the year 2004 for example, a poll conducted by HCD Research, revealed that 3 out of 4 medical doctors (of the 1,100 respondents who participated); believe in divine intervention, in the form of miracles.

I have personally read books by Thyroid Patient Advocates (proactive patients who help to inform fellow-patients), who include chapters in their books that encourage seeking spiritual as well as medical help for the emotional symptoms of thyroid disease.

I feel this is not an improper thing to do at all and in-fact, I personally believe that faith brings more hope to those who are seeking recovery and a better quality of life, in the midst of suffering medical health conditions.

Over the past few years, I have corresponded with other patients, who also expressed their Christian faith to me and I have derived much of the information within the chapters of this book, from my responses to their questions and their requests for advice regarding emotional symptoms.

In addition to well-studied layperson medical advice that I will offer following, it is my sincere hope that the chapters of this book also help to bring spiritual comfort and encouragement to those who are suffering thyroid diseases that have presented them with difficulties in treatment or challenges with learning to cope with their hypothyroid or hyperthyroid conditions.

-Jim Lowrance

CHAPTER ONE

Coping with Chronic Anxiety and Panic Symptoms caused by Thyroid Disease

I recently received correspondence from a fellow thyroid patient who shared with me the fact that they were struggling with chronic anxiety symptoms as a result of their disease that included aspects of "unreality sensations", also referred to as "depersonalization and derealization". These symptoms of severe anxiety and panic are very real and they cause the one experiencing them, to have sensations of feeling unreal (depersonalization) or of feeling as if their surroundings or aspects of daily life have begun to feel unreal to them (derealization).

In the case I refer-to following, the thyroid patient with co-morbid anxiety, who contacted me, was experiencing unreality sensations also regarding their Christian faith and so being both a thyroid patient myself and of the Christian faith, I was able to offer them some advice from my personal experience with these same issues.

Before I share the information I gave this fellow-patient let me also add that during phases of unreality sensations, a person can actually question the reality of their lives and even their faith-beliefs. This phenomenon of anxiety symptom-manifestation is common and does not indicate true mental illness, with aspects of psychosis not actually being involved. They are rather "sensations" that do not lead to one actually losing touch with reality or to permanently changing their beliefs that are of great value to them.

It is an aspect of chronic anxiety that has been studied by mental health professionals for many years and while they understand that the trigger for these sensations is caused by "the fight or flight response" -- the natural anxiety mechanism, they are not certain as to why this particular type of symptom occurs in some anxiety disorder patients but not in others. The ability for anxiety patients to overcome unreality symptoms and to cope with any phases of them that might occur is usually very promising with the correct treatment or therapy and with ample time given for these to effect the needed improvements.

Following below, was the advice I offered to my fellow thyroid patient, regarding their chronic anxiety and unreality sensations, associated with their hyperthyroid disease (overactive thyroid gland): ---

"Unfortunately some people who experience the unreality symptoms and the "brain fog" that can go with it, can experience it for years. Mine was fairly prominent for two years and would manifest to a lesser-degree for several years thereafter. I now notice practically no phases of it at all. I do still see the brain fog aspect from affected emotions or that results from bodily fatigue, which rears its ugly head at times (feeling foggy -- lacking mental sharpness) but even that is mild and intermittent, compared to my previous experience with it.

The way to look at it is to realize that it took years to develop these type symptoms and it might take years to see full recovery from them, although you might actually see a significant degree of recovery much sooner.

The good news is that anxiety unreality symptoms and the symptoms of chronic anxiety in-general, **won't lead to anything truly harmful**; although they do affect quality-of-life while you are going through them (they can also be somewhat discouraging at times, which is a natural response). You need to remind yourself ever so often, that you have lots of time to see gains over these symptoms, while your thyroid disease is being treated and there's no need to rush it because slow gains are usually the ones you retain better and you can also develop other coping skills while you are seeing recovery from the anxiety symptoms. Some often come naturally, apart from therapy -- your mind and body know how to make adjustments.

Also recognize while you are experiencing this, that people around you -- sometimes including family members, can find it difficult to empathize with your symptoms, simply because they have not experienced them and cannot understand them as a result. A lack of understanding can sometimes come across to us as "not caring" but that's really **not usually the case**. It's simply natural for people around us to lack understanding of what we are going through -- it's <u>human nature</u>. We may be tempted to think that they don't care; when they actually do have genuine concern for our suffering but they are at a loss for knowing how to express it (I hope that made sense from the manner in which I expressed it).

I am very happy to answer your questions. I feel that God places people in my path at times and I consider the sharing I offer, to the best of my ability, as a ministry he has given me. I have actually corresponded with people who reached a point of not wanting to live, due to their anxiety and/or depression caused by thyroid disease.

God forbid that I not help them to the best of my ability.

Depression is a very common thing to occur co-morbid (along with) severe anxiety. So if you do have problems with depressed mood triggered by the anxiety, do realize that it will lift, as the anxiety diminishes -- that's pretty much a guarantee. If depression occurs as a condition of its own, apart from anxiety, the same treatment advice I'm sharing would apply for this type of mood problem as well.

If you need psychiatric therapy or medications, as you develop coping skills, **this is nothing to be embarrassed about or to be ashamed-of**. You do after all have a medical condition and many of them can cause emotional symptoms, while they are being treated.

I'm a thyroid patient as well -- my treated disease being autoimmune hypothyroidism (Hashimoto's thyroiditis causing an under-active gland). I've gone through phases of chronic anxiety and unreality symptoms with mine, especially early into the onset of it, which first manifested with a phase of hyperthyroidism (overactive gland). I can assure you, that with time you can see those symptoms diminish and much of the victory comes through simply understanding the symptoms and knowing that they are not harmful apart from placing restrictions on our enjoyment of life, although they are extremely unpleasant to experience.

As you know, while anxiety is very much a physical thing and can directly result from a medical condition, it has spiritual aspects to it as well (if one believes in both body and spirit).

While I don't believe our spiritual enemy directly causes our anxiety (the one the Bible describes as tempting and oppressing mankind), he does try to influence us in the midst of it, to feel discouraged or like we're being persecuted for something we've done wrong or that we have not accomplished, etc... That aspect of it, the Bible calls "the spirit of fear" and we are assured that God doesn't give that type of fear to his children (fear of reverence for sacred things are different and proper and is not in the same category).

"For God hath not given us the spirit of fear; but of power, and of love, and of a sound mind." (2 Timothy 1:7 KJV)

The phase of questioning things, including your faith can be a part of the depersonalization/derealization symptom-aspect of chronic anxiety. I know this not only because it happened to me but also because I have read this stated by many other anxiety sufferers over the past 8 years as I've studied the subject. It added a great deal to their worry and increased their anxiety/panic symptoms because they even began to question their faith, God's existence etc...
However, as you know, we have a very compassionate God and he understands what we go through at every moment of our lives. When something is connected to a physical illness that we certainly can't help but to experience, he knows this as well and he understands the struggle these things can cause us.

The Bible says that "he is touched with the feelings of our infirmities", which means that he, literally experiences them with us. This is difficult to understand, with he being God but the likely answer to this mystery, lies in the fact that he abides in us, according to The Scriptures.

He knows fully, every detail of what we experience (the very hairs of our head are all numbered).

"For we have not an high priest which cannot be touched with the feeling of our infirmities (referring to Jesus Christ)*; but was in all points tempted like as we are, yet without sin."* (Hebrews 4:15 KJV)

"But even the very hairs of your head are all numbered. Fear not therefore…" (Luke 12:7)

Just remember that that "freak out effect" that severe anxiety or panic episodes can cause is not unusual at all, in fact it is very common. It will pass given time and you will be a stronger person on the other side of it, even if that sounds impossible at the present. Just give yourself permission to experience it and don't battle with it because anxiety thrives on struggle. Just kind of flow with it and let those small gains in coping happen over time because they will accumulate into bigger gains as you go along.

Prayer can be a great help as well -- probably your greatest weapon as you learn to cope and to overcome disordered anxiety (anxiety that occurs disproportionately or out of context). When we don't feel the strength to resist or to battle something that negatively affects our lives and emotions, we can turn it over to God in prayer because his strength never falters and he will win our battles for us.

"Thus saith the LORD unto you, Be not afraid nor dismayed … for the battle is not yours, but God's." (II Chronicles 20:15 KJV)

"Fear thou not; for I am with thee: be not dismayed; for I am thy God: I will strengthen thee; yea, I will help thee; yea, I will uphold thee with the right hand of my righteousness. " (Isaiah 41:10 KJV)

I wanted to add these words of encouragement, with your being in the family of God (we are also called "the body of Christ" -- 1 Corinthians 12:27). Even your medical treatment will greatly lend toward anxiety recovery, given time and it's my belief that God helped and inspired mankind to develop medical and therapy methods, for help in healing of both mind and body. Even one of Jesus' original 12 disciples was a doctor and in the New Testament, Paul the Apostle refers to him as 'Luke the beloved physician' -- Colossians 4:14."

CHAPTER TWO

The Effects of Thyroid Disease and Related Emotions on the Physical Senses

During correspondence with a thyroid patient recently, they mentioned to me that they were experiencing strange effects in regard to their eyesight, that they felt were directly resulting from mood changes associated with their thyroid disease. This person also shared with me, the fact that their emotional symptoms were seemingly hindering their ability to pray and worship God as they wanted to. Following was my response to their request for advice regarding this symptom affecting their eyesight and the oppression they experienced when desiring to offer prayer and worship to God. ---

"Anxiety can cause bizarre symptoms that one wouldn't think should be connected to it. I personally used to see groups of shapes when I would close my eyes at night, during anxiety episodes and they would be perfectly uniform, like wallpaper and sometimes they would fly across my field of view, like a bunch of little airplanes. I also used to see little twinkle-stars that would light-up in one area of my vision and then disappear. Strangely, these would be a different color -- sometimes blue or red or yellow, etc... While that sounds quite strange -- almost like visual hallucinations, I posted about this several years ago on a thyroid forum, where I used to be a moderator and lots of other patients described experiencing exactly the same visual phenomenon. Knowing that, helped me to not feel as strange or alone regarding my bizarre anxiety manifestations, most of which are now a thing of the past for me.

It's also possible that you have mild manifestations of thyroid eye disease, which is basically inflammation in the optical nerves. It is more common in Graves' disease patients (autoimmune hyperthyroidism) -- the type you have but Hashimoto's thyroiditis can cause it to manifest in some people as well (in those with autoimmune hypothyroidism).

Continue to self-educate regarding chronic anxiety and its symptoms because that will be a major tool against your disordered anxiety. One day you'll look back and you'll be amazed at how far you've come toward coping and overcoming it, if you practice self-therapy and give it plenty of time to take effect (i.e. practicing relaxation techniques, stress reduction, healthy diet, exercise and self-education on anxiety disorders).

It might also help to write about your experiences and post on anxiety forums or even on content article websites. Some websites actually pay you for page-views your articles generate or they share Google Adsense revenue with writers, which can be an added incentive. Reading other anxiety disorder people's forum-posts and articles can help as well because it's nice to relate to shared experiences and to see that others relate to the same experiences you are having.

My own thyroid disease related anxiety improved from both using coping techniques and with my thyroid hormone treatment. My coping mostly consisted of learning not to fear the symptoms of anxiety, so that I basically didn't resist them at all.

I just kind of flowed with them and so with my not adding even more adrenaline to them, by freaking out or anguishing over the symptoms; they faded on heir own over time. This doesn't work as well for everyone but I would imagine that the vast majority of anxiety sufferers would have some degree of success with diminishing anxiety and some with completely overcoming it, simply by learning not to fear the symptoms of it.

Cognitive Behavioral Therapists for example, will actually tell their patients to try experiencing certain physical symptoms, purposefully (i.e. blurred vision, tingling in their extremities, muscle tension) and afterward describe how these made them feel and what actual dangers or consequences that they perceived would occur as a result of them.

If they have difficulty experiencing a certain symptom on-queue, the therapist might actually induce the symptoms purposefully, in some manner. If they have problems with hyperventilating and dizziness for example, they might have the anxiety patient take lots of deep breaths until they feel dizzy, or spin them a few times in a swivel-chair to induce these physical sensations, to demonstrate their harmlessness.

Other therapists will have anxiety sufferers to expose themselves to their phobia-triggers but very gradually (exposure therapy). If for example, they fear settings with groups of people involved (social phobia); they will have them walk a few feet at a time, into a restaurant or into a mall, to slowly overcome their fear of joining-in with groups of people.

All of these types of CBT and anxiety-coping methods are to show them that the symptoms and the triggers (with the exception of real dangers), are really not harmful at all, no matter how unpleasant they may feel. Some anxiety patients learn to practice these techniques on their own, as self-therapy and mental health professionals actually encourage this. Following, is a link to a PhD psychologist's description of how harmless panic attacks actually are, in spite of how severe they may feel physically or emotionally to those who suffer them.

Click here or type this online link into your PC browser: http://www.anxietynetwork.com/pdfear.html

Naturally, when you're going through the harsher anxiety symptoms, it's very hard to stay connected, fellowship-wise with God or to even pray as you would like because your attention is terribly diverted by them. I had a very difficult time feeling inspired to fellowship/pray at those times I was suffering chronic anxiousness or panic symptoms, which were sometimes fairly lengthy periods in my life.

I know for a fact that God understands when we experience these temporary hindrances to our faith due to medical or emotional conditions and it doesn't mean our relationship with him is affected (fellowship hindered but relationship intact). I hope that information helps and I know you will be back to your old self soon, including your fellowship with God, as you work on coping and recovery, with His help. You may need to give it considerable time and let the recovery happen as gradually as necessary. Slow gains are usually the ones we benefit from the most."

CHAPTER THREE

Which Brand of Thyroid Hormone is Superior for Treating Hypothyroidism?

This chapter is derived from an answer to a question posed to me by a thyroid patient who was asking if a better choice of thyroid hormone replacement would be the Armour brand of hormone that is available for hypothyroid therapy. They asked this question in expectation of therapy for hypothyroidism that would follow surgical removal of their thyroid gland, as treatment for Graves' disease-hyperthyroidism. I feel the advice is important to include as a chapter in this book, for added perspective regarding the treatment of hypothyroidism because better treatment results in improved emotional symptoms. ---

"I'm actually on Armour brand of prescribed thyroid hormone myself (135mg = 2.5 grains per day). My personal feeling is that both Armour and Synthroid can work well for treating a patient's hypothyroidism and it all depends on getting the T4 and T3 to the right levels and TSH suppressed, as reflected by monitoring blood tests. With Synthroid (and similar T4 brands), your body converts the needed T3 from the T4 but with Armour, T3 is already in it, so the body requires less of it via conversion. However, it will still make up the difference if it needs to, should the T3 still need increased a bit in the body.

Some people can't take Armour if they're allergic to porcine products (anything from pigs -- but this isn't common) or they may be Jewish and have decided to consume kosher products only.

Yet other hypothyroid patients are overly-sensitive to the T3 in hormone replacement drugs and it causes them anxiety reactions. They will actually feel slightly hyperthyroid shortly after taking the dose, with anxiousness, nervousness and possible panic type symptoms (a fact I have seen attested-to many times on thyroid patient forums).

If you think Armour will do you well otherwise and is possibly superior to Synthroid in your case (entirely possible), you should request that the brand be prescribed to you by your doctor (most doctors are accepting of patient preferences and opinions). Keep in mind that some doctors are literally anti-Armour biased and they feel Synthroid is better in 100% of cases (might be true in some cases but the opposite can also be true).

With total thyroidectomy (surgical removal of the gland -- "TT") or ablation of the thyroid by radioactive iodine (I believe TT is the better choice), to treat autoimmune hyperthyroidism (Graves' disease -- overactive gland) you can go through several weeks of adjusting to hypothyroidism that develops afterward (under-active gland) and to the hormone replacement therapy for it that follows.

In the long-run however, it is definitely the right thing to do for the improved health of a hyperthyroid patient, as you have scheduled by the recommendation and referral of your doctor.

I would also add that praying over your daily replacement hormone dose, before taking it, can also add benefit to it in my opinion.

204

It is a common practice for us to pray and to offer thanks to God for meals we eat and I feel we should do the same over prescribed medications we are required to consume. I mention this; in light of your testimony in regard to being a professing Christian and I hope this advice has been helpful."

CHAPTER FOUR

Giving Thyroid Hormone Therapy Adequate Time to Work

In the response I am adding to this chapter, that follows below, I offered advice to a thyroid patient who reported that they were struggling with emotional symptoms, in spite of treatment for hypothyroidism via hormone replacement therapy and correction of sex hormone imbalances. They were only treated for a period of three weeks at the time they corresponded with me. An important fact I pointed out, is that it requires ample time for a daily thyroid hormone dose to result in the proper effect of restoring bodily metabolism and in correcting physical and emotional symptoms (usually several months). ---

"Some thyroid patients struggle a great deal with anxiety and panic symptoms resulting from abnormal fluctuations in their metabolism. I have experienced them myself and I know how very unpleasant they can be.

Lots of things can serve as triggers for anxiety attacks, such as endocrine hormone disorders including thyroid, adrenal and sex hormone imbalances. It sounds like you are being treated for these conditions that have been diagnosed, so getting added help for the anxiety itself can also be important, if it is causing you a struggle with coping. As you know, drug and psychiatric therapies can help, while your thyroid hormone dose becomes better optimized, should these become necessary.

Following is a list of psychotropic medications that are prescribed commonly for anxiety and/or depressive disorders:

Benzodiazepines for Anxiety:

• alprazolam (Xanax®)

• clonazepam (Klonipin®)

• lorazepam (Ativan®)

• diazepam (Valium®)

• buspirone (Buspar®) (this one is a azaspirodecanedione class drug)

Antidepressants for Anxiety and/or Depression):

• paroxetine (Paxil®)

• venlafexine (Effexor®)

• fluoxetine (Prozac®)

• setraline (Zoloft®)

• fluvoxamine (Luvox ®)

I would suggest conducting an online search regarding the side-effects and contraindications of these medications (potential adverse reactions and possible effects when combined with other treatments).

Most doctors are willing to switch their patients to a trial of a different drug, if one has been tried and the results are not satisfactory.

One type of psychiatric therapy that can also add great benefit is called "Cognitive Behavioral Therapy" (CBT) and is a highly successful treatment method. You can inquire with a doctor about referral to this type therapy or search online to find programs you can order for use at home as self-therapy. I personally benefited from several CBT programs I found online some years ago, so I suggest conducting a search using the name of the therapy and you'll find available programs that you can compare and take advantage of as a supplemental or mainstream therapy (leaving other treatment options open should they become necessary).

I do suggest however, that you inquire into programs that have the endorsement of mental health professionals or organizations. I have written several books on the anxiety disorder subject myself but none are actually CBT programs. They are more-so educational sources regarding anxiety disorders, symptoms and treatments that are available. I do however discuss aspects of CBT treatments in them, in some detail and I describe medical conditions that can cause or contribute to emotional disorders. I also discuss lifestyle changes that can effect positive change in mood problems.

You might also consider joining an anxiety forum (lots of these are available online as well) because reading fellow-sufferer stories and coping-success stories can be very helpful.

Gaining the knowledge that severe, generalized anxiety and panic attacks as unpleasant as they are, are typically not harmful or dangerous, although extremely unpleasant can lend greatly toward coping with them.

Do be sure to continue to get those extra helps for the anxiety as needed (i.e. prescribed medications and psychiatric counseling) or even as a permanent regimen if necessary because it is certainly nothing to be ashamed of if you require them for successful coping.

For a time I was on an SSRI antidepressant for anxiety and panic but I was weaned off of the drug, when my thyroid hormone therapy reached a level that really helped me and that adequately resolved my hypothyroidism. Sometimes it only takes months or sometimes it can take years to see treatments fix endocrine problems fully, that they are designed to address. Knowing that they will definitely effect the needed improvements over time, can give patients being treated that added hope that lends toward better coping.

The three weeks you mention being treated with thyroid hormone replacement therapy, is not nearly long enough to see the results you will eventually realize from the treatment. It takes about 8 weeks for a dose to become leveled-out in the body but even with this, you may need several dose adjustments (most likely increases) in your thyroid hormone medication, before you will reach an adequate or optimal replacement level.

In the U.S., the better thyroid-specializing doctors like to get the TSH blood level down to a 1.0 or a 2.0 (TSH elevates to levels above 3.0 with hypothyroidism).

They want the T4 level increased to above mid-range (T4 and/or T3 decrease to abnormally low levels with hypothyroidism) but the T4 does not need to be elevated too-close to highest-normal values, for concern of inducing "hyper"-thyroidism -- also referred to as "thyrotoxicity".

My honest opinion is that you will see more results from the hormone therapy as time goes on and as your dose is tweaked to a better level for you. Correcting hypothyroidism will definitely affect positive results with your anxiety and depression but if you need the added help of other medications or therapies, as previously mentioned, these are certainly options to consider.

Some hypothyroid patients can wean-off psychotropic drugs (antidepressants) once their hormone replacement takes them to a euthyroid state (normal thyroid levels) but this should be determined by the treating doctor via input by the patient and supervised by him.

I really do believe you will see better days ahead given adequate time on your thyroid hormone dosing."

CHAPTER FIVE

Healing Comes in God's Timing and Wisdom

I wanted to add a final chapter regarding more about my own case of treated hypothyroidism, which includes some of my related Christian testimony. ---

About mid-year in 2002, I was driving in my car and as will happen to me infrequently (not often), I heard words being spoken to me inwardly, that were authoritative and very clear. I'll describe what these words revealed to me in the paragraphs that follow below. First let me say as a Christian man, I fully believe in the leading of God in the lives of those who have accepted the salvation and Lordship of Jesus Christ and also for those he is leading toward salvation. That's everyone in my opinion and is something I believe to be stated in the Holy Bible.

"The Lord is not slack concerning his promise, as some men count slackness; but is longsuffering to us-ward, not willing that any should perish, but that all should come to repentance." (2 Peter 3:9 KJV)

I believe for most of us and most of the time, God leads us through our conscience by the Holy Spirit if we are open to it. There are times however that God may also lead us through supernatural words that come to us as a powerful inward witness. Some Christians have also been led by God with audible words at times and in Bible scriptures a number of examples of this can be found in both the Old and New Testaments. God doesn't change and he continues to speak to his people and to lead them today, just as he has always done in the past.

A Significant Event

Words that came to me inwardly were very much as powerful as those that could have been spoken to me in a voice I could hear audibly and pointed to a very significant event in my life. While I repeat this often in articles, I'll also say again in this book-chapter, that these type supernatural "words of knowledge" or "words of wisdom" (I Corinthians Chapter 12) have not been a frequent event in my life but when they do occur, they are unmistakable.

Like most Christians, I have for the most part experienced God's leading in my life through my conscience or what you might call an inward prompting. They are in a sense "gut feelings" that tell you what directions to go and decisions to make when you're willing and open toward listening to them. The Bible refers to it as "the still small voice" but it isn't quite the same thing as receiving specifically stated words that come through the Holy Spirit in a somewhat more powerful and supernatural way. This more simple leading is the Holy Spirit working through our own conscience.

I am a thyroid disease patient due to hypothyroidism caused by an autoimmune condition called "Hashimoto's thyroiditis". I had no reason previous to the onset of the disease, to believe I would ever experience a thyroid disorder of any kind. I did however receive a supernatural word in mid 2002 that gave me foreknowledge of the disease I was about to experience.

I cannot explain to you why some people experience more miraculous type manifestations or supernatural guidance than do others.

I certainly don't believe it is because God favors some people over others. Everyone is equally important to God and he loves us all the same and I believe this is clearly stated in his Word. I feel honored to have experienced these type things personally but if not another single supernatural type event happens in my lifetime, I'll believe God just the same as I do now and for the rest of my life. He will also continue to love me the same and lead me in those gentle ways if I will allow him to do so.

When this word came to me, I was not in prayer as I was at other times when similar supernatural words came to me, at other times in my life. I was simply driving my car and heard very plainly words spoken to me saying "your hormones are becoming imbalanced". As I've related in regard to other times I've experienced this type thing, it in-essence, completely stops you in your tracks so-to-speak. It grabs your attention in a major way because it is as if it is being spoken to you audibly and puts a feeling of total amazement and reverence in you because it is unmistakably real.

My only reaction at the time was thinking to myself that I barely knew what hormones were. I had scantly heard doctors on television talk about sex hormones and I had heard a little about adrenal hormones mentioned but my knowledge was very limited in this area. I had also heard a bit over the years about thyroid conditions but gave very little attention to it. Months later during that same year of 2002, I crashed into severe thyroid symptoms that phased back and forth between hypothyroidism (under-active thyroid) and hyperthyroidism (overactive thyroid).

I remember feeling terribly anxious and sweating profusely at night in bed, to the point of soaking the sheets I was laying on. The anxiety also began to escalate into full-blown panic attacks.

I still had no idea it was my thyroid doing this to me and when I went to the first doctor to describe my symptoms, I was diagnosed with emotional symptoms only (emotional disorder). I had not forgotten that word that came to me saying that my hormones were becoming imbalanced and my only question to the doctor was "could this be my thyroid?" Despite this question she would not order me blood testing, so I ordered them through another doctor's office. The results came back with two abnormal results on my thyroid panel and a follow-up blood test revealed autoimmune thyroid disease as the cause (i.e. positive and highly elevated TG and TPO thyroid antibody levels).

Suffering the Consequences of Man's Sin

Why did this happen to me? I may never know all of the reasons but I do know that I came very close to accepting the emotional diagnosis and I would not have demanded the blood tests and received a proper diagnosis and the treatment I needed, had I done so. I'm also a believer in God's supernatural healing power but I also believe God has a timing and wisdom involved in everything he does. We live in a fallen world if you believe the account of man's original sin, as recorded in the book of Genesis. The biblical record reveals man's choice to bring sin and the consequences of it into the world that God gave him dominion over.

This is why some of the negative things we see in the world today, are allowed to run their course and at times they affect our lives personally as well.

Other scriptures in the Holy Bible state that God will bring complete healing, deliverance and restoration to the earth he created for mankind but he will do so in his own timing and wisdom. In the mean time, those who go through negative experiences as I have with thyroid disease (there are much worse things), may have as part of God's plan a purpose in helping others who suffer the same problems. People often relate better in some ways to a fellow sufferer than they can even to their doctors or their own family members. They can also receive shared information and inspiration in helping others to better cope as they have learned to do.

Can Blessing come from Suffering?

In the early 1990s, I was miraculously healed of a severe stomach disorder that required prescription medications for many years to control the symptoms. I not only haven't received a healing in the case of my thyroid disease but I have also developed co-morbid conditions that I must also deal-with and be treated for.

I don't pretend to understand God's will completely on many things but I am certain that he at times takes things that are not yet fixed and uses them to bless and help others. It's not that they are necessarily God's will to occur but he sometimes takes things that cause pain and suffering and turns them into a blessing.

215

If we believe in the gospel story about Jesus suffering for others and his experiencing evil at hands of those who murdered him (he willingly laid down his life) we know that God may also use our experiences of suffering as limited human beings to bless others as he wills.

This has largely been the reason behind my passion for helping to educate and support others with thyroid disease. I'm simply a limited human being but to whatever extent I can help others, I feel it is an honor to do so and hopefully much of my effort is also pleasing to God. I'll always make mistakes along the way but with God's help and leading I will continue to do my very best.

I will conclude this final chapter, with a scripture regarding a physical ailment that was experienced by the Apostle Paul, who is considered by many Bible scholars, to be the greatest evangelist of the early Christian church (God inspired two-thirds of the New Testament, to be written through Paul).

While the scripture I will quote following, does not mention that God eventually healed Paul of his "thorn in the flesh" during his natural lifetime, it is my belief that he did receive a healing, that came within God's timing. Regardless, it is an inspiring scripture-passage.

We also know from other passages in the Holy Bible, that God does continue to provide divine health and healing, according to his will and wisdom (i.e. 1 Peter 2:24, James 5:14 and Mark 16:18).

2 Corinthians 12:7-10 (Apostle Paul):

"And lest I should be exalted above measure through the abundance of the revelations, there was given to me a thorn in the flesh, the messenger of Satan to buffet me, lest I should be exalted above measure.

For this thing I besought the Lord thrice, that it might depart from me.

And he said unto me, My grace is sufficient for thee: for my strength is made perfect in weakness. Most gladly therefore will I rather glory in my infirmities, that the power of Christ may rest upon me.

Therefore I take pleasure in infirmities, in reproaches, in necessities, in persecutions, in distresses for Christ's sake: for when I am weak, then am I strong."

(END - Section Six)

SECTION SEVEN:

Eighty-Seven Thyroid Disease Questions Answered!

Self-Educate through Hypothyroid and Hyperthyroid Q & A!

QUESTION ONE

Have you had Personal Experience with Thyrotoxicity - Overtreated Hypothyroidism?

Yes and I recently posted on a thyroid forum, in regard to being found in a state of over treated hypothyroidism. Following is my descriptive post in regard to this issue and how it is being resolved. ---

"Something has come up in the area of my hypothyroid treatment via Armour thyroid brand, combination - T4/T3 medication.

You will be blown away when you hear what my current blood levels are because I should be bouncing off the walls with hyperthyroid symptoms. Instead, I'm mainly fatigued, with stressed-out feelings. I do have muscle weakness and have been seeing a neurologist due to a few more sensory and tingling symptoms of aching, occasional stabbing pains etc... I had some low amplitude readings on an EMG but it's possible any nerve damage I have will be helped via the fact I was also found vitamin deficient in D, E and insufficient (low normal) in B12, which are all now being treated.

Now to my blood labs - (ready for this?)---

My TSH result was at "0.05" - Range 0.25 to 5.00 [TSH drops below normal with hyperthyroidism]

My FT3 was a whopping "903" - Range 210 to 440 [elevates with hyperthyroidism]

My Total T3 was nearly as bad (I prefer the free) @ "365" - Range 76 to 181 [also hyperthyroid level]

Yowzah! - Both T3s were more than TWICE the highest normal cut off value! In spite of this, my Dr.s Office called and said my levels were only "a little high" and in fact were going to place me on a DOSE INCREASE prior to seeing these results, because I have gained a little weight since my last visit and my T4 was actually on the low-side, which has been typical of how Armour manifests on my labs for the 7 or 8 years I've been treated with it. It was I who demanded my T3 be tested because they kept failing to add it on my lab requisitions, even with my repeated requests and I had a suspicion the levels were high.

Can a person have these high of levels and not actually feel like metabolism is sped up (hyperthyroid)? Regardless, I know it is very unwise to maintain this type level due to risk of bone loss and possible heart rhythm complications. I'm now also beginning to wonder if my high levels of T3 have contributed to my muscle weakness and peripheral neuropathy type symptoms (I know it is not the cause, since I began experiencing these symptoms long before the over-treated thyroid)!

In defense of the doctor, I will say that she had not yet seen the T3 result when she recommended the dose increase but based the idea on my T4 which was at "0.8" in the range of 0.9 to 1.8 ng/dL. My disappointment with the doctor is in the fact that a former MD I went to, who discontinued his practice due to a back problem, told me that T3 was important to test when taking Armour. I told the new doctor this at my first visit with her back in February, 2010 but she kept failing to add the test on my thyroid panels.

Treating Thyroid Disease Symptoms, Problems and Complications

I made sure it was added this time, by kicking and screaming a little and sure enough I'm over-treated.

I'm currently taking 2.5 grains, so will reduce it back to 2 grains and hopefully this will be enough of a decrease between now and when I get back in to a doctor (NOTE: I have since conferred with my doctor who agreed with the dose decrease and is monitoring it with follow-up blood retests)."

QUESTION TWO

Can Neuropathy and Myopathy Occur in Thyroid Disease?

The U.S.-NIH/NLM allows quoting of medical research published on their site (PubMed) for educational purposes and all of the quotes that follow below are from their site, with exception of the short quote I've added by the AAFP. I thought this might be of interest for hypothyroid patients like me. It shows that endocrine disorders in addition to diabetes are strongly associated with neurological disorders and symptoms.

(Note: In some studies, neuropathies did not resolve or only did-so partially in 'treated' hypothyroid patients and in my opinion, this is likely the case more often in "autoimmune" cases of hypothyroidism.)

(American Academy of Family Physicians):
"Muscle weakness is a common complaint among patients presenting to the family physician's office. Although the cause of weakness occasionally may be apparent, often it is unclear, puzzling the physician and frustrating the patient."

1. *Pain and small-fiber neuropathy in patients with hypothyroidism* (U.S. National Library of Medicine – PubMed) --- "Conclusions: Some patients treated for hypothyroidism have symptoms and findings compatible with small-fiber neuropathy or "hyper phenomena" indicating central sensitization. ...of Eighteen patients... Eight were classified as having large fiber neuropathy..."

2. *Hypothyroidism and polyneuropathy.* (U.S. National Library of Medicine – PubMed) --- "Using standard electrophysiological criteria, a definite diagnosis of polyneuropathy was made in 28 cases (72%). The commonest sites of abnormal nerve conduction were the sensory nerves, especially the sural nerve."

3. *Hypothyroid neuropathy and myopathy: clinical and electrodiagnostic longitudinal findings.* (U.S. National Library of Medicine – PubMed) --- "This case shows that thyroid hormone replacement eliminates the neuropathic manifestations of severe hypothyroidism. In contrast, the myopathic features, such as weakness and muscle wasting, may persist despite maintenance of the euthyroid state."

4. *Neuromuscular status of thyroid diseases: a prospective clinical and electrodiagnostic study.* (U.S. National Library of Medicine – PubMed) --- Among the thyroid patients, 17 (42.5%) patients were diagnosed with mononeuropathy and polyneuropathy. Entrapment neuropathy was observed in 30% and diffuse neuropathy in 10% of the patients. Myopathy findings were observed in 2 patients.

5. *Aspects of peripheral nerve involvement in patients with treated hypothyroidism.* (U.S. National Library of Medicine – PubMed) --- "RESULTS: Sixty-three per cent of the patients with 'pure' hypothyroidism had abnormalities on NCS, 25% had reduced IENF density and 31% had abnormalities on QST. Four patients (25%) met criteria for small fibre polyneuropathy, the other (75%) were classified as having mixed fiber polyneuropathy.

QUESTION THREE

Any Symptom Trouble Shooting Suggestions for Thyroid Patients?

I was diagnosed with Hashimoto's thyroiditis and hypothyroidism in 2003, at round about age-40. I do also have dysautonomia (imbalance in my involuntary nervous system) but I've never asked for a tilt-test (detects blood pressure imbalances that reveal dysautonomia) because I know for a fact it's there and has been since my teen years. I want to mention some things I had tested, that might give leads to fellow thyroid patients whose treatments failed to resolve certain types of symptoms they are experiencing.

Due to my unresolved fatigue, muscle weakness and neuro-type symptoms (despite treatment for hypothyroidism), one board certified MD suggested that I have comorbid (co-occurring) Chronic Fatigue Syndrome because I have apparent immuno-deficiency including allergies (i.e. thyroid autoimmunity and mild persistent asthma). In the case of CFS however, one must rule out all other possible causes of unresolved symptoms.

I believe, among many other things, one should have vitamin levels tested, such as B12, B6 and E because each of these can negatively affect the nervous system if deficient (as can low D) but the problem is usually easily reversed with supplementation of deficient vitamins. I was found deficient in D and E and insufficient (low normal) in B12. I had my doctor test me for kidney/liver levels and anti-mitochondrial antibodies (AMA), to make sure my malabsorption was not due to kidney or liver problems.

I do have fatty liver (I'm moderately overweight) but no biliary involvement or hepatitis (serious liver diseases). It doesn't hurt to rule these out if one is diagnosed with deficiencies of fat-soluble vitamins (ones previously mentioned).

Also, this is another suggestion to discuss with a qualified doctor but "thyroid antibodies" can be present/positive before thyroid hormone levels become imbalanced, so if these haven't been tested-for, this might be something to also consider if one is experiencing unexplainable symptoms. According to the U.S. NIH (PubMed), thyroid antibodies can cause symptoms even when the person affected is in a euthroid state (normal hormone levels).

I also feel that symptoms can also point to the need for a person's sex hormones to be tested and these can be affected if adrenal hormones are low, such as pregnenolone and DHEA which convert into sex hormones (both androgens/male and progesterones/female, which both sexes have in different balances) as the body needs them.

I personally also have adrenal fatigue - also since 2003 or earlier and repeat saliva and urinary cortisol tests showed mine to be low but DHEA was always normal or even high-normal. Adrenal saliva test kits can now be obtained through local pharmacies or online. I've always felt that lack of immunity (immune system dysfunction), dysautonomia (nervous system imbalances) and endocrine dysfunction (problems in hormone-producing glands) are all tied closely together. One imbalance of a system can affect one or all of the others. These are just a few suggestions for trouble-shooting unresolved symptoms in treated thyroid patients.

QUESTION FOUR

We Know Hypothyroid Treatment is not perfect but is it Essential?

I'm one of the rare male hypothyroid patients with Hashimoto's thyroiditis. Just this year, I was finally tested for vitamin deficiencies and my D was also deficient at: "17" ng/mL (range 30 to 100). My B12 was lower-normal, so I'm treated for both it and the D with replacement mega-dose vitamins.

I went to a neurologist-specialist due to long-term muscle weakness and easy fatigability - that I was convinced since 2004, was CFS (chronic Fatigue Syndrome), comorbid to my thyroid disease. He had the forethought to also check my vitamin E, since my D was deficient and B12 was insufficient and "Presto!" it was deficient as well, at: "0.4" (range 3.0 to 15.8) - in fact, at less than half a point was likely my worst deficiency.

I've been active as a patient advocate since diagnosis and my 'sometimes' difficulty with some doctors - such as my current over treatment on thyroid hormone replacement for hypothyroidism (my blood work showed my T3 to be more than double highest normal range). ---Little things like that (LOL).

Anyway, I mainly try to dispel the imbalanced opinion (kindly, diplomatically and politely) that suggests that thyroid hormone replacement is perfect in all cases and fixes all the problems thyroid patients have within weeks of being administered.

Don't get me wrong - I thank God for thyroid hormone therapy and for doctors but without patient proactive ness in their treatments, things can most certainly go wrong, regardless of a doctor's expertise or a thyroid hormone brand's effectiveness. There can also be comorbid (co-occurring) disorders like vitamin deficiencies or a number of other things that also need to be diagnosed and treated.

So---- My message since 2003 to other patients is to become self-educated, best possible, via good, reliable sources and to be proactive in treatment and to partner with their doctors if at all possible!

QUESTION FIVE

Any Association between Dysautonomia and Thyroid Disease?

I believe there is and I'll give my personal experience as an example:

I have had orthostatic hypotension since my teens, mine being the type that only causes me the weird pressure sensation in my head and neck due to a short episode of blood pressure drop when I first stand-up but I've never had syncope with it (fainting). Rarely when I was younger I would experience the drop-out of my vision for just a couple seconds. In-short, with my other symptoms of chronic fatigue, generalized anxiety etc..., I believe I'm likely in the POTS (Postural Orthostatic Tachycardia Syndrome) or MVPS (Mitral Valve Prolapse Syndrome - common heart murmur) category.

I also have Hashimoto's/hypothyroidism, which I understand to be a common finding in dysautonomic patients and in those with MVP and in the past few months I was found deficient in 2 vitamins (E and D) and insufficient/low-normal in a third one (B12) - all being treated. I also believe due to my symptoms for many years of heart skips, flutters (less frequent than they used to be) and extreme sensitivity to caffeine, chocolate and alcohol, that I also have Mitral Valve Prolapse, even though my EKG was normal in 2001 (was having frequent symptoms then). I've not had an echocardiogram - sound wave imaging of my heart but don't really feel I need one to confirm MVP because it runs in my family.

I just had EMG/Nerve Conduction studies done this year (2010) due to worsening of carpal tunnel and tarsal tunnel type problems and general muscle weakness. Part of this is likely a result of my vitamin deficiencies but because of my tendency toward anxiety/worry I became neurotically concerned about having ALS, MS or some other terrible disease. I will say this in regard to that fear about my muscle weakness, that I've had it far too long to be caused by a neuromuscular motor neuron disease, unless it is the slowest developing, least-aggressive type. I can remember posting on forums about my muscle weakness in 2004/2005 and these posts still exist out there somewhere. I actually remember as far back as 2002 having these same type muscle symptoms and my thyroid treatment that began in 2003 never resolved them, leading me to think I had comorbid CFS (Chronic Fatigue Syndrome) to my hypothyroidism. I have never seen any atrophy in my muscles.

QUESTION SIX

Can one be Over-Treated on Armour Thyroid Prescribed Hormone?

I was recently found to be over-treated on thyroid hormone replacement therapy as I stated in an earlier answer to a similar question, which is sometimes referred to as "dose induced throtoxicity" (hyperthyroidism). The following was my giving detail to this problem in a forum post. ---

Strangely enough, I didn't have classic thyrotoxic symptoms like tachycardia/rapid heart rate or weight loss (in fact I have difficulty losing - moderately overweight) however, I can't imagine it not having affected me in some way because my last blood retest for T3 was as follows:

FT3 result - "903" (range 210 to 440) ----[This was twice highest normal + 23!]
Total T3 result - "365" (range 76 to 181) --- [twice highest normal + 3]

Before this, I was kept at highest normal on T3 and occasionally, just slightly above normal but TSH was always kept at near undetectable, such as "0.005".

The reason I agreed to this dose-level for about 6 years is because my T4 will actually drop slightly below normal if my TSH even rises to between 0.5 and 1.0. I felt this indicated that I instead needed some T4 added rather than increasing the Armour but none of my doctors would agree to do so, claiming it makes for too much opportunity for instability of the treatment.

I had even thought years ago about switching to T4 but I feel that patients used to getting T4/T3 combo, need to continue it or risk falling into symptoms by switching to T4 only (i.e. depression) or their bodies may be slow in converting T3, due to it having been supplied for so long. Certainly this might not be the case but was something I didn't want to risk.

This is not a knock at doctors in-general, I assure you but in the area I reside-in, finding good doctors is an incredible challenge. I've heard many other people in my area express this same opinion - so I'm far from alone in it.

I got to post regarding this to the board certified endocrinologist at the other thyroid forum and will be eager to see if he believes my myopathy (muscle weakness) might be related to the over-dosing. I'm also treated for D and E vitamin deficiencies and feel these play a factor as well but I certainly don't want an additional cause or contributor to that symptom!

Once seeing my Armour over-dose levels via blood retests, my Dr. had me cut back from 2.5 to 2.0 grains of the prescribed hormone and said she will blood retest me in 3 to 4 months but even this seems like a strange timing, since I feel 8-weeks would be better, so that it can be adjusted even further if-needed.

[NOTE: The MD at "the other thyroid forum" I mention above, did confirm to me, that over-treatment with thyroid hormone, can indeed cause or contribute to myopathy (muscle weakness)]

QUESTION SEVEN

What is the Importance of Thyroid Test Normal Values Ranges?

The following was my response to a fellow thyroid patient who was found to have a very low TSH level via blood tests. They also had a T4 test done (a major thyroid hormone) and a T3 Uptake (not a measure of the T3 hormone level and usually only useful in diagnosing thyroid disease). I mention in my reply to them, that posting results of blood tests is more useful for getting comments on, if the normal values reference ranges are also included. ---

"Your TSH is near undetectable and decreases to low levels with hyperthyroidism (overactive thyroid). Your T4 test might be flagged high as well but if you could post the normal range for comparison that would help.

The T3 Uptake is not always helpful but if you could also post the range for it and the FTI Index, this would also help since labs differ in normal values ranges.

If your doctor is having the thyroid ultrasound done, this is to see if you have abnormal textures in your gland or nodules (small tumors) that can cause your thyroid to overproduce hormone if they are "hot" - meaning they are acting as if they have become thyroid tissue - absorbing iodine and manufacturing, putting out excessive amounts of hormones.

The other tests he ordered (mentioned but not detailed in your post), I'm willing to bet are "thyroid antibodies" ones, to see if the cause of your hyperthyroidism is autoimmune (Graves' disease). The antibodies he ordered might include the TPO and TSI, the later mentioned being "Thyroid Stimulating Immunoglobulin" - the ones typically found in Graves' disease. He might also be ordering a test of your T3, which is not listed above. T3 Uptake doesn't measure the T3 hormone level but measures how well the blood uptakes T3 hormone via available binding globulins."

QUESTION EIGHT

Are Non-Prescription Thyroid Glandular Supplements Available?

Most of the thyroid glandular products have the hormones extracted from them because this is the only way they can legally sell it non-prescription. You might read their ingredients to see if this is the case. Also, if it contains iodine, this will not successfully convert into thyroid hormone without your gland present to complete the conversion process (if it is diseases or has been removed). This means the iodine could possible build in your system over time (not a certain but a possibility) and this can cause a degree of iodine-toxicity if it goes too high.

On the other hand, if you monitor the effects of the supplement closely and ask your doctor for copies of your repeat blood tests of thyroid hormone levels, this too can help tell you if the supplement is interfering with your hormone replacement therapy (if being administered) or if it is actually aiding it.

I'm a believer in natural supplements but in some cases when you require hormone replacement for which there is no substitute, they can hinder the therapy. No two cases are exactly the same and each patient can be different in this respect, so using the safeguards I mention above (monitoring) can help determine if the supplement is helping or hindering.

QUESTION NINE

Is Determining the Cause of Hypothyroidism Important?

According to medical research, some cases of Hashimoto's thyroiditis (common autoimmune cause of hypothyroidism) do not present with positive antibodies tests but will be detected by Fine Needle Aspiration (thyroid tissue biopsy).

Here's one source that mentions this:

"Hashimoto's thyroiditis: fine-needle aspirations of 50 asymptomatic cases."
Viral thyroiditis and sub acute usually present with hyperthyroidism (overactive) and resolve within a few weeks and are not followed by hypothyroidism. Analysis of a thyroid tissue sample would be differentiated by a reviewing specialist.

Supplements that contain high levels of iodine have been shown to contribute to thyroid autoimmunity resulting in either Grave's disease (autoimmune hyperthyroidism) or Hashimoto's thyroiditis in some people who take them.

If the cause is not within the gland itself - primary, it can be a secondary cause. Since there are many possible causes, including secondary ones such as other disease processes going on in the body, age-related (if elderly), thyroid regulating brain gland problems (Central Hypothyroidism), etc..., it may take considerable testing and a process of elimination to find a definitive cause.

Many Dr.s aren't too concerned about "cause" they simply treat the under active thyroid and if treatment improves it, they call it good. Most patients do however want to know the cause if at all possible (some Dr.s do too), simply to know what's going on in their bodies.

I recently heard from a man, who wrote me in regard to developing hypothyroidism after he had been taking an herbal supplement, that he felt triggered a case of thyroiditis in his thyroid gland. It is possible that the supplement the man had been taking was causing the hypothyroidism and stopping the herbal might have corrected it. It's hard to imagine that it would have caused permanent damage unless thyroid autoimmunity resulted from it or there was some other agent in it that caused damage to the gland. People vary in their tolerance to herbal supplements, so anything is possible.

In my opinion as a layperson - non medical professional, the T4 and T3 hormone levels should be blood tested to see if only the T3 is lowering in new cases of hypothyroidism that have no cause determined for them. This can happen with "low T3 syndromes" like Wilson's Temperature Syndrome and Euthyroid Sick Syndrome and in cardiac patients.

QUESTION TEN

Is Vitamin D Deficiency and Thyroid Autoimmunity Connected?

Vitamin D deficiency has been found in medical research to cause immune system problems. There have been studies showing that it places people with both deficiency (blood-level readings of 20 ng/mLand below) and insufficiency (blood-level readings of 30 ng/mL and below) at risk for autoimmune disease and other chronic and inflammatory diseases, including those affecting the thyroid gland. My reason for researching on the D deficiency syndromes, is due to my personally being diagnosed with deficiency (my result was "17 ng/mL"), which I'm currently being treated for. I have Hashimoto's thyroiditis caused hypothyroidism and I now have yet another possible cause of mine - vitamin D deficiency.

Autoimmune thyroiditis very rarely goes into remission or I should say rarely reverses but is usually life long and replacing low vitamin D levels is very important but will not cure the disease either. So far no treatments have been found to cure autoimmunity of any kind although patients with Graves' disease can see hyperthyroidism permanently resolved with thyroid removal or ablation with radioactive iodine. They do afterward have to be treated permanently with thyroid hormone replacement. One thing that does help reduce thyroid antibodies (the immune cells that cause the disease) according to med-research is supplementing with selenium at the recommended dose on the label. Other than this, there's no cure for the thyroid autoimmunity itself. I wish there were because I would get it administered for mine.

Some sources I went to, to search about Drisdol (my prescribed treatment for D-deficiency) state that it's a "D2" replacement vitamin. I looked at my prescript bottle and it says Generic for: DRISDOL - which I had not noticed before either. It does state on the label: "50000UNT" - The mfg: "BRENC" (apparently an abbreviation for the company). Some sources state that deficiency needs to be treated with "D3" rather than D2 for better improvement. I'm going to be retested on my 25(OH)D level in a couple months and at regular intervals of about once a year, thereafter. If I remember correctly the blood test shows both D2 and D3 levels (I get copies of all labs I have done). While my original deficiency reading was "17" as mentioned previously, even a level of 30 is considered "insufficiency" and I believe they like to see the level increased to at least 50 or above. If this Vitamin D brand doesn't get my levels corrected properly, as reflected in follow-up blood retests, I will definitely ask for a change to D3 supplementation.

QUESTION ELEVEN

Increased Anxiety Symptoms with Hypothyroid Treatment?

This article is my response to a thyroid patient who underwent Radio Active Iodine destruction of their thyroid gland (RAI Ablation) and upon becoming hypothyroid following; they were started on replacement hormone therapy. The new hormone dose was causing some bodily adjustment symptoms of anxiety and following was my response to them in regard to this. ---

I'm sorry to hear you are struggling with the anxiety. I've been there and now how terribly unpleasant it can be! Mine did improve greatly and I believe yours will too, over time. It's hard to be patient when you feel miserable but I would encourage you that with your ongoing treatment and blood retests, your doctor will know how to adjust your replacement dose of thyroid hormone.

Once you are better leveled-out, which can take some time following radioactive iodine treatment (the thyroid ablation you mentioned having), you'll see the anxiety symptoms improve.

It's a strange phenomenon because it can actually cause hypothyroid therapy to induce even more anxiety at first but once you are on a proper dose of prescribed hormone, you should see the anxiety symptoms improve after a few months (maybe as little as 8 weeks).

239

When I say proper dose, many reputable thyroid specialists believe TSH needs suppressed down to "1.0" for patients to see optimal symptom improvement.

In my case, it took a few months after I was on proper thyroid dose to see my anxiety symptoms improve significantly. Mine did actually increase for a while, especially during the first few weeks on my initial dose.

QUESTION TWELVE

Can Anxiety Symptoms Occur with Taking a Thyroid Hormone Dose?

This article was my response to a hypothyroid patient who wrote me in regard to experiencing anxiety symptoms while adjusting to a new dose of replacement hormone therapy. ---

I can relate to what you are going through. The first doctor, who treated me, placed me on a full replacement dose of thyroid hormone (Synthroid), when most doctors like to start at a lower dose and build it up to full-replacement. It kicked in very strong anxiety symptoms that literally made me pace a circle in my living room because my resting heart rate went up to about 150 and I was hyperventilating. Once I was on a stable, correct dose for about two months, the anxiety resolved for the most part.

Yes, both too low a dose and too high a dose can cause anxiety symptoms. A low dose causes your body to try compensating for lack of thyroid hormone by increasing adrenaline, which is the same thing that happens to hypoglycemic people when their blood sugar/glucose goes too low. A dose that's too high causes anxiety for obvious reasons, because the metabolism is being spiked too much, too quickly.

Thyroid hormone therapy is a delicate balance but some doctors don't approach it that way and think any reading that's within normal values is good. The fact is however, that some patients need a sustained optimized level of hormone in their body.

241

It could be that given a few more weeks, your current dose will adjust better in your body because it usually takes 8-weeks or so for this to happen. I will have to say that I'm surprised your Doctor does not see the importance in retesting your blood level to monitor the new dose and if he still doesn't agree to do so within a few more weeks, I would find a doctor who is willing. If you're still walking around with an imbalanced thyroid level, this needs to be determined or it needs to be confirmed that the level is good. Blood levels are the most accurate way to know if you have good levels or need an adjustment to them.

QUESTION THIRTEEN

What do Positive Thyroid Antibodies Mean?

The positive thyroid antibodies blood test means you have autoimmune thyroid disease. Your doctor will likely do further testing, if not already, to determine if you have Hashimoto's thyroiditis, which causes hypothyroidism (under active), or if you have Graves' disease, which causes hyperthyroidism (overactive). This will depend on what a thyroid panel shows - whether your thyroid hormones are decreasing or increasing as a result of the antibodies attacking/attaching to your thyroid gland. You didn't mention which type antibodies were found positive but if it was the TPO or TG ones, this would point to Hashimoto's if your thyroid hormones (T4 and T3) are low and/or if your TSH is found to be high (elevated). The opposite will be true of these (low TSH & high thyroid hormones), if Graves' disease is the case.

First Hashimoto's can be diagnosed no matter how long you've been on thyroid hormone. They detect it via the "anti-TPO" and "anti-TG" antibodies tests and I would bet big that yours would return positive on either or both. As your Doc to order these because it will only take him a stroke of the pen to do so.

Some believe the 'cause' of hypothyroidism isn't important but I feel a patient has a right to know if it is autoimmune (hashi's) because autoimmune diseases place you at slightly higher risk for others like diabetes and rheumatoid arthritis.

As per your question as to what type of doctor I prefer for my own health provider needs, an Osteopath (D.O.) is actually my preferred Dr. because they believe in a degree of natural supplements, in-balance but do not go as far with it as naturopaths do (Note: there is no substitute when prescribed thyroid hormone is needed). D.O. physicians also require more education than do regular MDs/GPs and they can be just as board certified as any other MD and can deliver babies, perform surgeries and prescribe medications.

QUESTION FOURTEEN

Any Medical Research Available on Anxiety and Thyroid Disease?

Lots of medical research states that autoimmune thyroiditis can cause anxiety symptoms and even anxiety disorders in some patients.

Here are some quotes in regard to this:

" In a study of patients with Hashimoto's thyroiditis, anxiety was a prominent initial symptom at the time that the condition was diagnosed." (Richard Hall MD PhD - Johns Hopkins) -
LINK>
http://www.drrichardhall.com/anxiety.htm

"The study seems to suggest that individuals in the community with thyroid autoimmunity may be at high risk for mood and anxiety disorders. The psychiatric disorders and the autoimmune reaction seem to be rooted in a same (and not easy correctable) aberrancy in the immuno-endocrine system." (U.S. NIH) -
LINK>
http://www.ncbi.nlm.nih.gov/pmc/articles/PMC516779/

"We have found that sub clinical thyroid dysfunction increases the anxiety of patients whether hyperthyroid or hypothyroid." (U.S. NIH) -
LINK>
http://www.ncbi.nlm.nih.gov/pubmed/15256776

245

These studies quoted above, are not even in regard to yet another condition that can occur with thyroiditis called "Hashitoxicosis" (intermittent or temporary hyperthyroidism), which can occur in some patients before progressive hypothyroidism sets-in.

"Hashitoxicosis is a transient hyperthyroidism caused by inflammation associated with Hashimoto's thyroiditis disturbing the thyroid follicles, resulting in excess release of thyroid hormone." LINK>Hashitoxicosis - Wikipedia, the free encyclopedia

These sources make it very clear that anxiety can occur with autoimmune thyroiditis.

QUESTION FIFTEEN

Are There Side-Effects Adjusting to a New Thyroid Hormone Dose?

Thyroid hormone replacement takes about eight weeks for a new dose to fully adjust in the body and to begin doing its job. Treatment can take longer however, depending on how many dose-adjustments are needed to get you to adequate/optimal levels. Many patients need one or two adjustments because Dr.s often start at a low dose and increase it upward which is called "titrating the dose". You should see more symptom-resolution as more weeks go by.

All types/brands of prescribed thyroid hormone are designed to take over the thyroid gland's production, which is inadequate when hypothyroidism is present. As the hormone comes in from outside of the body, the pituitary gland (in the brain) senses the increase in the blood stream and sends less TSH to the thyroid gland (Thyroid Stimulating Hormone). For some hypothyroid patients, they will experience a break-even point, before improvement from increasing thyroid hormone levels begins to occur.

Also: Many medical research articles also attribute hypothyroid symptoms to the "thyroid autoimmunity" aspect of thyroid disease, rather than just to the abnormal or fluctuating thyroid hormone levels but some doctors aren't aware of this fact.

QUESTION SIXTEEN

Is there a Need for Synthetic and Natural Thyroid Hormone?

I've read articles in regard-to how, in the early days of treating hypothyroid patients, they fed them raw animal thyroid glands. The patients usually did very well on this strange method of treatment. Just the fact that thyrotoxicity (treatment-induced hyperthyroidism) happens with taking too high a dose of thyroid hormone replacement (patients testify to this happening today), is why safeguards are in place. Is the system perfect? As you and I know, of course not. When patients don't respond favorably to the standard treatment, doctors need to look at every single area of the replacement to see if it can be tweaked (adjusted for improvement) even more. If every avenue has been explored in improving a patient's treatment, including exceeding the optimal dose (as agreed on between Dr. and patient), only then, should other causes for unresolved hypothyroid symptoms be looked into.

I am one of those patients that didn't do well on Synthroid, synthetic T-4 only medication and was switched to Armour brand – natural T4 and T3 combination and began doing much better. My mother however has been on Synthroid for many years and has done very well, with no need for switching her brand. When I mentioned Armour to her several times, asking if she thought she might do even better, she refused to inquire with her doctor about it because of feeling so well on the Synthroid and didn't want to upset the applecart so to speak (why try fixing something that's not broke?).

I have read that some people actually have the opposite effect happen to them - they have bad reaction to Armour and are switched back to a synthetic brand (either T4 only or a combo T3 and T4). Some people for example, are allergic to porcine products, pork etc.... If Armour (made from pig thyroid glands) was the only brand available, what would happen to these hypothyroid people needing treatment?

Is Armour superior in treating hypothyroidism? For some people it absolutely is superior and extremely-so, in some cases. This may be true in a majority of cases but synthetic still needs to be available for people who need another option, including those who cannot take the brand due to their religious affiliation, requiring kosher observance (consuming no pig by-products). A patient's excitement and pro-activeness in advocating for a particular thyroid hormone brand, is a good thing and may someday contribute to causing reform of those things in regard to hypothyroid treatments that aren't good (i.e. treating according to lab ranges only, with no consideration for unresolved symptoms). This is true of those who advocate for synthetic brands as well.

QUESTION SEVENTEEN

What's the Difference between Optimal versus Over-treated Hypothyroidism?

I am on 120mg (2-grains) of Armour brand - thyroid hormone replacement therapy. I was first placed on Synthroid three years previous to my Armour dosing and my Dr. switched me due to concern I was one of those patients who have problems with T-4 to T-3 conversion (impaired conversion). As far as my having been on the dose I described in an earlier article that suppressed my TSH to 0.006 (far below normal), I was on that dose for several months, which placed me at risk for become toxic on the thyroid hormone (TSH goes lower as thyroid hormones rise in the body). My intermittent joint and fatigue symptoms did not improve but the fatigue worsened dramatically after I had been on the higher dose for about three months.

As far as heart problems at hyperthyroid levels (hyperthyroid is used interchangeably with hormone-toxicity) and many other serious problems it can cause, I'll give you a first hand example of what hyperthyroidism, regardless of cause, can do to a person. --- My Uncle had Graves Disease and became hyperthyroid as a result. It was not treated for too long of a period and in addition to dramatic weight loss, he developed a heart aneurism, needing corrected by surgery and he also experienced a stroke from delayed treatment of the hyperthyroidism. The reason Dr.s equate thyroid hormone toxicity (also called thyrotoxicosis), with hyperthyroidism, is because it can have identically the same effects on a person.

Treatment-individuality of patients on hypothyroid therapy needs considered, I agree, which is why symptomatic treatment, without TSH testing/monitoring cannot be safe for every patient. One reason is because with some people, the line between thyrotoxicosis (over-treatment) and being asymptomatic can be a very fine/thin line.

Also, my unresolved symptoms, that I attempted to resolve by increasing my thyroid hormone dose, were almost certainly not thyroid related (I was later found to have 3 vitamin deficiencies). You may remember in Mary Shomon's book "Living Well With Autoimmune Disease", she states that with her thyroid medication dose optimized, she had lingering symptoms and was also diagnosed with co morbid CFS/Fibromyalgia. She takes low-dose antibiotics to relieve her joint pain and on her Thyroid-Info website she stated in an article, that at one time she went off the antibiotics and the joint pain/fatigue returned. I do not know she still requires an antibiotic or if she was able at some point to discontinue them.

My opinion is that a well treated thyroid condition can still have co morbid conditions existing with it (medical sources state that 25% of patients with thyroid autoimmunity can get other autoimmune diseases). My belief is that there are subtle viral infections, allergies etc... that can cause symptoms as separate entity-illnesses. I for example, have low cortisol levels but not Addison's disease (Adrenal Fatigue). In fact, I had a cortisol test result recently, of "1.7" in a normal range of "3 to 8 ng/mL". Not only does thyroid hormone not treat low adrenal conditions but it can actually lower cortisol even further in people with varied degrees of adrenal insufficiency, which means it is separate issue, needing separate attention.

ALL THINGS cannot be linked to thyroid but I certainly believe thyroid patients need to be optimized to the best possible levels on their thyroid hormone dose that also does not place them at risk for over-treatment. Thyrotoxicosis from over-replacement is a genuine possibility. As far as the question of whether I have actually heard of people going hyperthyroid from over-replacement - Yes, I have seen people's testimonies of this many, many times on thyroid info websites and message boards.

QUESTION EIGHTEEN

Any Opinions on the Thyroid Stimulating Hormone Blood Test Debate?

I would like to express something about the TSH treatment-level debate (Thyroid Stimulating Hormone – blood tests). First let me say I sometimes (for lack of a better term), "play dumb" when I inquire about a subject on thyroid patient discussion-forums, so that I get unprompted opinions and so that I'm not leading an answer I might get, in the direction I want it to go. When I tell someone I agree with them, I may be speaking about a specific, not a blanket agreement on everything.

Second, I want to admit, the suggestion about suppressing TSH (elevates with hypothyroidism) to almost undetectable levels before some patients experience symptomatic relief, led me to finally experiment in this area, with my own medication, which I strongly and emphatically DISCOURAGE anyone from doing. I did-so because of desperation for symptom relief from ongoing joint pain flare ups and severe fatigue spells. I do some contract work requiring a lot of physical stamina and I need a certain amount of wellness, to keep going. I very slowly increased my thyroid hormone medication, above that recommended by my Dr., until my TSH was almost undetectable. I did not have any hyper/toxicity symptoms but experienced a severe, bone numbing fatigue, which means I likely was at the edge of dangerous reactions to the dose. My symptoms did not improve. I am now at the dose-level originally recommended by my Dr., with a TSH between 0.5 to 1.0.

My opinion is that "certain" people have a pituitary response (gland that sends out TSH in response to thyroid hormone levels) that is sluggish but not actually at the "hypopituitarism" level (under-functioning pituitary gland). Their Free T-3 and other levels can be upper, but not top-normal and their TSH will already be suppressed to near undetectable level. The problem is - how can a Dr. assume someone is in this category, when the majority of people are not? This is why a standard is set that covers the majority of people treated for hypothyroidism. Most Endocrinologists and thyroid specialists, even the AACE (American Association of Clinical Endocrinologists), recommends a treatment TSH level below 3.0, so the goal of 0.5 to 1.0, is even more optimal. To narrow it even further, is simply too risky for the majority of people.

Hyper-toxicity (thyrotoxicity) from over-treatment (hyperthyroidism induced by too high a dose) can actually be life-threatening and no-one should want to see that risk taken on wide scales but only with those individuals who apparently have the slight pituitary abnormality and need a little more attention. These people need repeat testing of their other hormone levels besides TSH. I think what happens is that someone who does obtain optimal symptom relief by symptomatic adjustment of their thyroid hormone dose, rather than by using the in-range cautions, believes their experience proves this success goes for everyone who might attempt this and they are understandably very excited about it. In reality, the majority of people need a TSH level at the low-normal cut-off range or can be at very serious risk for things like heart arrhythmias and chronic bone loss (osteoporosis).

QUESTION NINTEEN

Does Polyglandular Autoimmune Disease Occur in Thyroid Patients?

There are complications that can off-spring so-to-speak, from autoimmune thyroid disease (Hashimoto's thyroiditis). Diabetes is one of them but patients are practically never informed about this. I know this from corresponding with 100s of fellow patients over the years, since 2003. Some of the diseases that can develop in people with autoimmune hypothyroidism are "Polyglandular Autoimmune Diseases" and there are two categories of these. One type is a combination of Hashimoto's and Addison's disease (adrenal insufficiency) and they also refer to this one as "Schmidt's Syndrome" or "PGA I". The other is a combination of several diseases such as Hashimoto's with adult onset diabetes (type II), adrenal insufficiency and hypo-parathyroid disease - a dysfunction in the endocrine glands that regulate calcium levels in the body. When these glands become either hyper-functioning (high) or hypo-functioning (low), they can cause symptoms similar to hypothyroidism. This other type of polyglandularproblem affecting several glands in the body is referred-to as "PGA II".

Dizziness upon standing (Orthostatic Hypotension) is a major symptom of low adrenal function, especially when you experience it severely enough to actually pass out from episodes of it (syncope). They usually check your cortisol (cortical) levels and for adrenal antibodies, to rule out or diagnose the presence of adrenal dysfunction/disease.

They may also test to see how well the adrenals respond to being stimulated; via the "ACTH Stimulation Test". The other co morbid disorders that can occur with autoimmune thyroiditis, are detected via testing for imbalances in these other endocrine glands, if they suspect that problems have developed in them.

QUESTION TWENTY

Treatment Options for Hashimoto's Thyroiditis?

From what I have read on many medical sources, many people are found to have Hashimoto's Disease, when their hormones are all within normal-range. I'm sure you know this but for sake of those who might not and are reading this, Hashimoto's is an autoimmune disease with no cure and causes hypothyroidism at different rates of progression. Some people have it for many years before having symptoms. Other people are discovered having it, along with a goiter (thyroid swelling) being the only initial, physical symptom.

Other medical information I have read state that the autoimmune attack that causes this common form of thyroiditis causes symptoms in some patients even before hypothyroidism sets-in but the majority of Dr.s do not believe this. Be prepared that if you suggest treatment be started for you (unless you have a more informed Doc), that he/she will likely tell you, you're having emotional problems not related to your thyroid disease because after all "your other labs (apart from positive antibodies) are within normal range".

I hate to say it but I am so glad my TSH and T-3 Uptake were both out of range, indicating hypothyroidism, on my very first blood tests. I didn't have antibodies checked-for until 2-years later because the Doctor I was seeing wouldn't order them for me. When I did have the tests performed, both my TG and TPO ABs were elevated.

I had terrible anxiety symptoms, mixed with depression for MONTHS before getting that first test and even though I told my Doctor at that time that I felt it was my thyroid causing symptoms, she prescribed an anti-depressant, Xanax (anti-anxiety drug) and a beta-blocker to treat my symptoms, rather than testing me for treatable thyroid hormone imbalances. My symptoms worsened as a result.

When I finally demanded that first blood test, they failed to notify me regarding results, so more than a month later, I called the Doctor's office, asking "where's my test result". They said; "sorry it must have gotten lost for a while but there is nothing on the report indicating anything needing treatment." I then called the lab itself and asked for a copy, which they were able to provide, via my signing a release. I had two abnormal readings on the thyroid panel (High TSH and Low T-3 Uptake), plus elevated cholesterol (another sign of hypothyroidism). I took the results to a new Doctor and he placed me on thyroid hormone replacement medication even though he said "it's only a sub-clinical case of hypothyroidism". Since then, I've had four dose increases of my hormone drug and may have more to come in the future (now on 150mg – Armour).

I would certainly research about thyroid removal or oblation (RAI killing off the thyroid) before going through with it for your Hashimoto's thyroiditis (it is usually restricted to cases of Graves' disease – hyperthyroidism). You will basically have the same result letting your gland die out more gradually through the antibodies process. You will need full replacement once it is removed, with thyroid hormone medication, following the procedure.

I don't know if all people who undergo thyroid removal have to have dose adjustments or not or if some are given a full replacement dose that is started and maintained, with little or no adjustment needed (it likely varies with each patient).

I would research about all possible post-effects of that ablation procedure before I would have it done but I also wonder if a Dr. would even seriously consider it, without your lab ranges being more outside of normal values or without severe thyroid pain occurring in your case. I believe Hashimoto's patients can have fluctuating symptoms also due to life events (stressors) and the same is true of Graves'-hyperthyroidism. The reason I believe this is because people with proper functioning thyroids, will have it adjust automatically to extra mental stressors and extra physical activity, that obviously place more demand on their bodies for increased thyroid hormone levels. With hypothyroid patients, we are on a set-dose of replacement hormone, so that we are operating on the same amount no matter what extra demands are placed on our bodies due to emotional/physical stress, illnesses, etc...., which is why adequate replacement dose-levels are so important.

Again, I would suggest researching your treatment options and discuss them fully with your doctor, including asking about risks involved, should you be offered the option of ablation (radioactive destruction) or removal of your thyroid.

QUESTION TWENTY-ONE

Any Comments on Diagnosing and Treating Autoimmune Hyperthyroidism?

Derived from a forum post I wrote in 2005. ---

When I mentioned "borderline" (in reply to your post) I only meant on the TSH reading you were bordering on being flagged low. Borderline just means right on the edge of being abnormal (TSH drops low with hyperthyroid conditions). As far as the condition itself that you might have causing over-active thyroid, only complete testing can reveal if it's full blown Grave's disease (autoimmune hyperthyroidism) or if it is just entering that phase of abnormal for some other reason. You are right about antibodies being the test to see if the hyperthyroidism is autoimmune or not because there are secondary causes of hyperthyroidism, such as a pituitary gland that puts out too much TSH, due to a tumor within it (rare) etc...however, your TSH is low, so that probably rules out the pituitary as your cause of over active thyroid.

If you have elevated antibodies along with hyperthyroidism (especially the "TSI" ABs), that pretty much reveals the cause right there, as being "Grave's Autoimmune Hyperthyroidism". Blood tests will reveal if it's autoimmune and there's also the possibility of either or both a goiter or nodules (small tumors in the gland). Goiter is thyroid swelling and nodules are small growths, common in both hypothyroid and hyperthyroid patients with autoimmunity as the cause.

Sometimes it's good to get a second opinion. I did this back when I was struggling with Hashimoto's Disease (autoimmune hypothyroidism), trying to get diagnosed and coincidentally, it was the thyroid antibodies test that actually finally told me what was causing my hypothyroidism. I too got second opinions in my case and never told my regular Dr. because I felt it was none of his business unless I completely switched to a new doctor and needed my medical records transferred.

Your current Doctor seemed to think the only treatment was to remove or ablate (destroy via radioactive iodine), part of the gland but that is usually only done, in milder cases of hyperthyroidism, if medications don't control symptoms. Do you have high blood pressure or tachycardia (rapid heart beat)? If you do, it is strange that she isn't concerned about it as a complication of your abnormal increase in metabolism. Maybe your symptoms are mild enough, that she doesn't want to consider these other medications at this point but your mention of panic attacks made me think your vital signs might be operating high. Xanax might calm down your nerves but not sure it would help with the hypertension and high heart rate (tachycardia). Your case definitely needs investigated further and followed-up on and you might consider that second opinion by a qualified thyroid specialist or endocrinologist.

QUESTION TWENTY-TWO

Should Doctors Consider Hypothyroidism Symptoms versus Lab Results Only?

It's always disappointing, hearing about a Dr. that won't treat a patient who has severe symptoms of under active thyroid, just because their lab ranges aren't out of range enough yet. I believe you said antibodies were already found to be positive in your case (per your post). That means your thyroid hormone "receptors" can be blocked by the antibodies, causing hypothyroid symptoms, even with hormone levels in normal range, according to some medical websites. Also, the antibodies can cause development of goiter and/or thyroid nodules (tumors – usually benign) and thyroid replacement medication can halt this or reduce already existing ones in the gland.

Some Dr.s who treat hypothyroidism are "lab-range only" ones and others look at these other issues listed above and other types of symptom-manifestations to determine the timing of starting a patient on treatment.

Some Dr.s claim it is their concern over making a patient go "HYPERthyroid" if they treat too early and that this can cause osteoporosis and heart arrhythmias however, why can't they reassure against this through follow-up blood testing, just like with other patients on treatment for hypothyroidism? Websites I've researched claim that the osteoporosis possibility has been completely blown out of proportion and does not occur easily, unless a patient is severely over treated for long periods of time. As far as heart arrhythmias go, if they begin to occur, a Dr. might simply reduce the dosage slightly, to alleviate them.

You might consider a second opinion if a doctor is reluctant to treat mild but symptomatic hypothyroidism but make sure you take all lab results with you and always get copies of all labs each time tests are completed.

I personally would never use herbal methods to treat a thyroid disorder. I believe people who do, are playing with fire! You need Dr. Supervision and blood testing follow-ups for hypothyroidism to be treated properly.

I get very passionate about bad Dr. Treatment but I have EVERY CONFIDENCE in the good ones out there, of which there are many. There are plenty of good, quality physicians but the trick is in finding them.

As to the antibodies, there is no cure for them and they cause a disease process in the thyroid gland that is most often life-long. They have to run their course although thyroid hormone replacement medication may significantly lower the antibodies levels over time in some patients. SO THERE is another positive reason for starting thyroid replacement medication in patients with the autoimmune type disease in their thyroid glands.

The antibodies will keep attacking until there's no more living thyroid tissue left to attack and so a patient who is not yet at a level of hypothyroidism that requires treatment, will reach that level at some point – some sooner than others.

QUESTION TWENTY-THREE

Can Antibiotics Aggravate Thyroid Autoimmunity?

Antibodies from the immune system are natural and produced by the body and are specific toward the invader they need to attack. It's amazing how the body can make these toward whatever needs eradicated, such as allergens and bacteria's we are exposed to. Antibiotics on the other hand are micro-organisms produced by man, for administering to people with infections caused by bacteria but they are ineffective against viruses.

Could antibiotics attack antibodies that go against one of our organs? This I don't know, does anyone else out there? There is supposedly an antibiotic that a select few people have taken and it cured their Hashimoto's thyroiditis but I will not believe this until I see it announced on reputable medical sources (would be nice though).

I really don't believe there is any chance of antibiotics increasing thyroid antibodies, one they are administered to someone to treat an infection. They are actually two different things and I believe they would continue to do their separate jobs, although we don't like the job the thyroid antibodies are doing in cases of autoimmunity in the gland (disease process). I don't think there is any danger at all in people with thyroid autoimmunity taking antibiotics and I'm sure Hashimoto's patients are placed on these type drugs as often as anyone else. You might however, want to tell a Dr. or Dentist that you have Hashimoto's, when they suggest antibiotics or any other medication, just as a precaution, to see if they believe there could be any adverse interactions (contraindications).

QUESTION TWENTY-FOUR

Does Thyroid Disease cause Emotional Symptoms?

This article is derived from a forum post I wrote in 2005.

There is a very definite problem with Doctors telling patients their emotional problems are not due to their thyroid disorders, when the patient knows for fact it is. They believe a person only attributes the emotional issues to thyroid because they don't want to admit an emotional problem. EVERYONE has a certain degree of anxiety and depression, at times, or they are not human because these are natural emotions but thyroid disorder people develop more problematic type emotional problems and they know for a fact it came with development of their thyroid condition.

The second Dr. I went to after I was diagnosed hypothyroid, I asked; "Can hypothyroidism cause anxiety & depression"? He replied; "No, only tiredness." After he told me this, I got online and went to website-after-website by reputable medical sources and every one of them listed "depression" as one of the most common symptoms of hypothyroidism. Many of them included "anxiety" as a symptom as well. Other websites, containing lots of personal stories by hypothyroid patients, commonly had them mentioning anxiety along with the depression that was caused by their thyroid condition. Why do some Doctors want to see the emotional symptoms as not being related to the thyroid condition, especially when they are not completely relieved by treatment?

Who knows for sure but I do know they are relentlessly pushed by pharmaceutical companies, to mass prescribe antidepressants and Doctors themselves often admit this (I heard one refer to this recently on a radio program).

If a thyroid patient does not have adequate dose of thyroid medication and this causes symptoms to linger, why not let an optimized dose be reached and given a chance to relieve symptoms before an antidepressant is prescribed? This has always been my question in light of the increasing frequency of antidepressant prescribing to hypothyroid patients who are inadequately treated on thyroid hormone. If a thyroid patient complains that their symptoms haven't been relieved as expected, the first thing a Dr. should do is check to see if they need a dosage increase of their hormone replacement therapy because Hashimoto's patients commonly develop a need for dose increases due to the thyroid gland progressively dying-out (atrophy).

QUESTION TWENTY-FIVE

Is Combining Antidepressants with Hypothyroid Therapy Okay?

I was placed on an antidepressant when I went to a Doctor feeling ill and I finally weaned slowly off of it when I requested my own blood lab tests and it was found that I had autoimmune hypothyroidism.

Let me say; I believe antidepressants can be very helpful to people and I personally know people who are on them and doing great. The reason I personally got off of them is because my root problem was not emotionally caused, it was thyroid disease caused. I wanted treatment for it before I considered an antidepressant, so that I would not confuse thyroid symptoms with the drug side effects. Some of the antidepressant side effects are; "fatigue, lightheadedness, dizziness, sexual dysfunction, nervousness, tremor", etc.... – the same as are listed for thyroid hormone imbalances.

PLEASE UNDERSTAND, I am not suggesting that anyone quit taking the antidepressant they are prescribed, what I am saying is; If you find through lab testing that you have hypothyroidism, you need to get treatment for it, in addition to the antidepressant because an untreated thyroid disorder can be worsened with antidepressant treatment alone. SSRI antidepressants can lower thyroid hormones even further, when one has autoimmune hypothyroidism, according to research I have read, so can affect the need for dose adjustments in thyroid hormone treated patients.

Many medical sites state this but one study I can refer to in particular is one from Sept., 2004, conducted by "UCLA School of Medicine, Dept of Endocrinology" THEIR CONCLUSION: "With Antidepressant treatment, the most common change in thyroid hormones is a DECREASE in T-4 and Free T-4." That study tells me, if you have hypothyroidism, an antidepressant can potentially make it worse if left untreated and unmonitored.

QUESTION TWENTY-SIX

Is There Importance in a Qualified Thyroid Doctor?

I know there are top-notch thyroid Doctors out there but they are becoming rare. If you can get in to see a specialist for thyroid disorders, I would certainly consider it.

Dr.s sometimes use the psychosomatic (emotional) explanation for unrelieved symptoms of treated thyroid disorder, when it is a difficult case. This of course is possible with any patient and any disorder but I personally do not believe it is the case with as many patients as they seem to believe it occurs in. I say this because I personally know people who were under-treated for their thyroid disorders plus have read testimonies of hundreds of others, who were told their symptoms were mood-related or imagined. How can this many people be having imagined or emotionally caused symptoms? Common sense tells me it is related to their thyroid disorders and they need more specialized care.

My last two Doctors were Endocrinologists and still gave me strange advice, so you need to check references etc... to choose a good one that is genuinely qualified in thyroid treatments. Examples of things I was told by my Endo-doctors; "Your TSH is on the edge of high-normal (elevates with hypothyroid and the goal of treatment is suppress it) but since it is within the reference range, your symptoms cannot be thyroid related" and: "You have Autoimmune Hypothyroidism but is probably only temporary (actually it is lifelong in vast majority of cases)." ---

And: "It is extremely rare to have adrenal insufficiency or another autoimmune disease with Hashimoto's thyroiditis (some medical source state that 25% of patients develop co morbid health disorders, much of it being other autoimmune diseases).", etc.....

The fact is; The TSH has to be low-normal, not high normal, for a hypothyroid patient to feel better on thyroid hormone replacement. ALSO; Hashimoto's requires life-long treatment with hormone replacement and people who have experienced remission of the disease are the ones who are "extremely rare". ALSO; One in four (25%) of Hashimoto's patients develop other related disorders as referred above. The above is why I say you might need a second opinion from a qualified specialist, in case you were misdiagnosed or are not getting optimal treatment.

Under treatment for thyroid patients is way too common and will take people like us to help make a difference, through patient advocacy (sharing our experiences and self-educating). I sometimes wonder if Doctors are required to update their knowledge in thyroid treatment protocols, since so many new things have been learned over the past several years. If not, we really can't place full blame on the Doctors who are not being updated via available avenues. Maybe new requirements for updates to Doctors should be enforced, so that inadequate treatment cases can be reduced.

QUESTION TWENTY-SEVEN

Is There Varied Effectiveness of Antidepressants in Thyroid Patients?

From a forum post I made in 2005. ---

If I remember right, I think you said on a past post, that you had a high TSH on your blood tests. From what I understand Grave's disease never causes an elevated TSH but a suppressed (low) one.

Hashimoto's patients do have hyperthyroid, Grave's type symptoms commonly, I know I did for a good while and at first thought it was just severe anxiety. A Doctor placed me on Paxil for a few months too (SSRI Antidepressant), a few years ago but for me personally, I couldn't stand the side effects of the drug. I got really trembly and weak in my body (already had some of this but it became worse). I also had electric "zap" type sensations that went from my head, all the way down to my toes. Not to be too personal, but it also affected my libido (sex drive), causing a significant drop in it.

Some people may do well on these type drugs but I didn't. It took quit a few weeks for me to completely feel free of the lingering build-up of the antidepressant in my system, when I weaned off the drug very slowly with my doctor's help. Please don't let this be a discouragement to anyone out there because as I said, some people may benefit a great deal from SSRI-Antidepressants but I am one patient who didn't.

271

I'm glad you SLOWLY came off the antidepressant,
because some people stop them abruptly (bad idea) and for
some reason, most Dr.s don't warn about this or tell
patients about the side-effects and severe withdrawal
symptoms from not gradually tapering off.

Your hyperthyroid symptoms should improve over time
and your hypothyroid symptoms as well but it takes a lot
of patience as you better adjust and receive any necessary
dose-adjustments.

QUESTION TWENTY-EIGHT

Do Hyperthyroid Symptoms occur from Hypothyroid Therapy?

ALL thyroid medications have the same potential to cause heart arrhythmias and is really a matter of taking too much of any of them, that can cause this (same warning on all of them applies). I too take Armour brand but first was placed on Synthroid. I was just the opposite, I didn't have arrhythmias but I had HYPER-thyroid type symptoms when I first started Synthroid. When I was switched to Armour, I never once had these symptoms.

I've read that some people are more sensitive to the Armour brand (natural T4 and T3) than to the Synthroid (synthetic T4). I believe this is because Armour (made from pig/porcine thyroid glands) has both hormones in it and medical researchers say T-3 has more potential to cause hyper type symptoms such as arrhythmias than the "T-4 only" medications do. Even your TSH reading of 1.0 (approximate rage O.5 to 4.5) would seem good because they recommend as low as 0.5 for some people with stubborn hypothyroid symptoms. Yes, you can go from hypo to hyper thyroid with autoimmune thyroiditis and many on this forum have attested to this. I too, early on, had really severe anxiety and waking up during the night in cold sweats etc... Mine finally went to progressive hypo and stayed there but occasionally I do have some anxiety symptoms. Medical websites I've researched say both hypo and hyper thyroid patients can have it as a manifestation of thyroid autoimmunity, regardless of corrected hormone levels.

As far as hyper swings, then back to hypo, it is due to the antibodies attack against the thyroid and its response while it is able, in releasing large spurts of hormone to compensate against damage being done to it. We, in a sense have germ warfare going on in our bodies you might say! You'll see on medical sites that Hashimoto's thyroiditis patients commonly have hyper swings until the gland is so damaged it can no longer fight back against the immune system attacking it with auto-antibodies.

QUESTION TWENTY-NINE

Can Thyroid Hormone Therapy cause Adjustment Side Effects?

This article is derived from a forum post I made in 2005.

It's good to see you on here on the forum again but I am sorry it is because you are not feeling well (per your post). I too had worsening of hypothyroid symptoms after starting thyroid hormone replacement medication and I was so disappointed because I knew just the opposite was supposed to happen. On many of the websites I've researched, they talk about the introduction of medication with many patients, actually causes the thyroid to atrophy (cut back it's own production of hormone), so that even though you are putting hormone into the body from the outside, for a while you only break even, or even lose ground with your levels.

Sometimes it takes more than just the few weeks that they blood-retest a patient, for this altered level-change to show up. The TSH is suppressed immediately because there are more thyroid hormones (T4 and T3) in the blood stream but by the time the body actually utilizes that extra hormone, the levels start dropping again and a dosage increase is needed all over again! Others on this post have experienced this, as I have too and are even now getting increased on their dosages. It is very frustrating because the process seems so to take so long!

275

Your breathing trouble could be pressure on the trachea from swelling of your thyroid, according to what I have also read or could just be hypo-lack of thyroid hormone (oxygen hunger), slowing down your vital signs. I do know that the constipation alone CAN MAKE YOU FEEL SICK. In fact you need to keep trying to find a solution to it because it can become toxic at some point if it becomes severe. This happened to a nephew of mine and he became ill due to it. Your symptoms, including the constipation, certainly do sound like hypothyroidism. Given time however and proper dose adjustments, you should see better days ahead, soon.

QUESTION THIRTY

Can Chemical Sensitivities happen with Autoimmune Thyroiditis?

The brief article following was a forum reply I made to a thyroid disease patient who found that they had negative aftereffects from consuming alcohol. ---

Thyroid disease does cause increased chemical sensitivities in some patients; in fact they call it "Multiple Chemical Sensitivities" (MCS). I know since having Hashimoto's, I have extreme sensitivities to caffeine and chocolate. I always had some sensitivity to these but it worsened with thyroid disease. It could be you had a more severe reaction to alcohol (per your post) because of your thyroid. I also have sensitivity to alcohol, which I found out kind of inadvertently. I drink very occasionally (infrequently) and in June-2005, my wife and I celebrated our 22nd anniversary with a bottle of Champagne (rare for us). I admit I finished-off the bottle because it was not a large size and had low alcohol content for a wine product and I started feeling sick afterward, which lasted several days! In my old days, before I reformed (LOL), I could drink most people under the table. I'll never do those things again, since becoming a Christian, plus I have no desire to become intoxicated on chemicals of any kind but I know for certain that reaction I had was a result of the thyroid disease, among other possible factors involving health disorders I have co morbid to my Hashimoto's thyroiditis. Conditions such as adrenal fatigue, Mitral Valve Prolapse (heart murmur) and Chronic Fatigue Syndrome can cause MCS as a feature of them as well.

QUESTION THIRTY-ONE

Any Personal Experience with Adrenal Fatigue Co-morbid to Thyroid Disease?

When I was diagnosed with hypothyroidism, my readings according to the Doctor were only "sub clinical", with a TSH of "8.3" (range 0.4 to 4.8) and a T-3 Uptake flagged "low". The rest of my thyroid hormone levels were in the lower half of normal. It wasn't until two years later I got the thyroid antibodies ones tested and my TG ABs were "537" (normal being <40)and my TPO ABs were "84" (normal being <35), so this was the test that actually confirmed Hashimoto's thyroiditis (autoimmune hypothyroidism).

ANYWAY, here was my problem from the beginning; after I started my thyroid hormone replacement medication, some of my symptoms actually WORSENED. I was frustrated, so did a search using "Worse symptoms after starting thyroid replacement medication" (or something to that effect) and it took me to sites stating; If you have UNTREATED adrenal insufficiency, this can worsen if you start thyroid hormone medication. This was also stated on the thyroid brand maker's websites! I decided I would get checked for "cortisol" levels, it being the "major stress hormone" that regulates glucose and stress-levels in the body, among other things! I searched and found "Great Smokies Diagnostic Laboratories", who put out BodyBalance-StressChek Brand, home saliva tests to check DHEA/Cortisol levels. These are as accurate as blood tests, according to medical research groups.

My DHEA was about mid-range but my cortisol on 4-different ones of these I took over a year period, were all either low-normal, borderline low and one was clinically low. I then found another company that sets up blood testing for LabOne and I got a 24-hour urine cortisol test done. The range on the urine test was <119 for males age-18 and older and my result was "10.7"! I finally made it to an actual Dr. visit and showed him these readings. As I suspected, he patronized me a bit but went ahead and sent me for an "ACTH Stimulation Test" (Expensive for a self-pay patient but highly diagnostic).

I was VERY ANXIOUS when I had the test done, which probably gave a falsely high "baseline cortisol level". They first get your baseline or starting level, and then inject you with ACTH - the hormone, that stimulates your adrenals to produce cortisol. They then rechecked my cortisol at 30-min and 1-hour intervals. My baseline was "10.7", my 30-min reading was "25.7" and my 1-hour reading was "37.4". So, I passed the stimulation of my adrenals quit well BUT this DID NOT change the fact that my cortisol levels are low, without stimulation!

There is some reason for my low adrenal output of cortisol and I suspect it to be "adrenal fatigue", triggered by autoimmune thyroid disease. My symptoms have been; orthostatic hypotension (temporary dizziness/pressure in head when standing) slow resting heartbeat, low resting blood pressure, fatigue, joint pain, post exertion fatigue (after physical activity), all of which I originally attributed to my thyroid disease.

I do know that some of this worsened with my thyroid hormone medication treatment but I need it or risk worse hypothyroid symptoms that can result in severe consequences if left untreated. I have instead added adrenal support supplements when I need them, to help with times of symptom flares from adrenal fatigue that occur due to fluctuations of low adrenal cortisol levels.

QUESTION THIRTY-TWO

Are there Similarities between Overactive Adrenals and a Hyperactive Thyroid?

My reply to a forum post regarding: "Overactive Adrenals Versus Hyperactive Thyroid".---

ACTH (Adrenocortitrophic hormone) is the hormone the pituitary gland releases to stimulate the adrenal gland to release more cortisol, just like TSH is released by the pituitary gland, to stimulate the thyroid to release more T-4 & T-3. The problem is, that too-much ACTH, also means overproduction of cortisol, so that means your adrenal glands are overactive (Cushings Syndrome) when this is happening. That is why your blood and/or urine cortisol reading will be above the normal range. Your Dr. will try to determine if it is caused possibly by a tumor in the pituitary gland or other cause.

Don't let this scare you because just like a thyroid tumor (hot nodule) can cause the thyroid gland to overproduce (Graves' Disease), a pituitary or even adrenal tumor can also cause overproduction of the hormones they stimulate production-of (cortisol, ACTH, DHEA etc...).

If there is a tumor, it is very rare that it would be cancerous, just like it is rare for thyroid tumors/nodules to be cancerous. They usually control these imbalances with medication but of course only a qualified Dr. can determine this through further diagnostic testing.

So, in a nutshell, they want to reduce your elevated cortisol if it becomes elevated for the preceding described reason or for other reasons, which causes "Cushings Disease" symptoms (excessive cortisol levels). Do an online search to learn more about this by going to a search-engine and put in the term "Symptoms of Cushings Disease".

I personally had the "ACTH Stimulation" test administered (a measure of adrenal function), not just my "ACTH" levels measured (pituitary hormone that stimulates adrenal output of cortisol). My adrenals do under-produce adequate cortisol but not severe enough to be called "Addison's Disease" (opposite of Cushings), meaning too little cortisol, which does cause me symptoms of adrenal fatigue/exhaustion. I believe the medications they use to treat Cushing's patients are what they call cortisol-inhibitors but they do also try to remove any tumor they might find in the pituitary gland that is causing the hormone imbalance.

As far as thyroid tumors/nodules go, I think the reason most of the time, they don't remove them (unless suspected of malignancy) is because thyroid hormone is easier to replace if hindered by a nodule than trying to replace all of the hormones the pituitary is responsible for sending out to the other endocrine glands (hormone producing) in the body. Also, the kind of tumors that cause excessive hormone production are more dangerous than ones that cause inhibited hormone production such as in hypothyroidism. Tumors that Graves' Disease people have (overactive thyroid glands) do result in more surgeries to remove them than do the kind that are found in patients with Hashimoto's thyroiditis (under active thyroid glands).

They also sometimes "oblate" (destroy) the thyroid glands of Grave's patients because hyperthyroidism is more immediately dangerous, due to its effects in causing increased heart rate and blood pressure.

This is kind of the same problem with the Cushings disease, which is 'sometimes' more immediately risky than Addison's because it causes excessive hormone levels in the body. With Addison's, it is kind of like hypothyroidism - all they are required to do, is replace the low hormones, as determined by blood testing all levels that might be affected but with Cushing's (adrenal), as in Grave's (thyroid), they need to remove the cause of the over-production, so that damage does not occur to other organs in the body.

QUESTION THIRTY-THREE

Can Thyroid Disease Affect Speech?

From my forum reply regarding: "Can Thyroid Disease Affect Speech?".---

I'm willing to bet that sometimes people looking into this forum and others for thyroid disease support - maybe even Dr.s, who happen-by to read the postings, think that we are attributing too many things to thyroid disease but - here goes again! Some medical websites actually mention "difficulty pronouncing words", as a possible symptom of thyroid disease.

There is a woman who has an interesting website, her name is "Sonja Midtlien", she is Norwegian and if you will put her name into the search-bar of www.google.com, I'm sure her thyroid website will be listed, for you to click on and go to, for browsing/reading. She mentions that the "Norwegian Thyroid Association", lists "difficulty pronouncing words", as a symptom of Hashimoto's-Hypothyroidism and they state that the cause is "due to enlargement of the root of the tongue". That's their words, not mine, so everyone out there can take it for what it's worth! We do know our thyroid gland regulates EVERYTHING in our body (metabolism), so it would not be hard to believe that speech can be affected in my opinion.

QUESTION THIRTY-FOUR

Is Asking your Doctor for Thyroid antibodies Testing Okay?

From my forum reply Re: "Asking your Doctor for Thyroid antibodies Testing".---

If you find your results at home and don't see that they tested you for thyroid antibodies levels, I would ask them to add this to your future ordered tests when you can. I'm not telling you what to do, it's just a suggestion because many Doctors for some reason don't test hypothyroid patients for thyroid antibodies (The "Anti-Thyroglobulin and Anti-Thyroperoxidase") and these are the ones that tell you if it is autoimmune hypothyroidism or not. People with Hashimoto's thyroiditis (most common autoimmune cause in industrialized countries) have to monitor for any new sets of symptoms, worsening ones etc... because they are at increased risk for other autoimmune diseases, such as rheumatoid arthritis, adrenal insufficiency, diabetes, etc..., so if a Dr. says "it doesn't make any difference what kind of hypothyroidism you have or what is causing it", I would tend to disagree with him. In my opinion IT DOES MATTER what is causing a thyroid hormone imbalance and it's your body - you have a RIGHT to know what types of disease-processes are going on in it.

Sometimes Doctors make a patient feel a little silly, because they suggest a test, treatment option etc... but the Doctor-Patient relationship should be more open than that, so don't feel intimidated if your Dr. seems reluctant to work with you, in establishing a cause of your under active thyroid gland.

He may be the type that does listen, so I don't mean to pre-judge him (there are certainly many great Dr.s out there), I just wanted to prepare you for what most of us out here have been through in having to suggest or even sometimes "demand" that testing be ordered to further evaluate our thyroid disease cases. We refer to this as being a "proactive patient" and studies have shown that activated patients are the ones who get better treatment.

QUESTION THIRTY-FIVE

Can Hashimoto's Thyroiditis cause Anxiety and Depression?

From my forum reply regarding the question - "Can Hashimoto's Thyroiditis cause Anxiety and Depression?".

Yes, you can have both anxiety and depressive symptoms with hypothyroidism, especially if it is the autoimmune type (Hashimoto's Thyroiditis). Most of us on this forum can relate to this because we have experienced this. Sometimes I'm concerned that it always sounds like I'm knocking Dr.s and I really don't mean to come across that way but some Dr.s believe that just because your lab ranges are normal on blood retests you have done to monitor your thyroid hormone therapy, that this means you should also feel "normal". The fact is however, that progressive hypothyroidism that has an autoimmune cause (i.e. Hashimoto's thyroiditis) can make you swing back and forth between hypothyroid and hyperthyroid symptoms, including aspects of low mood and anxiety and sometimes these episodes even become mixed.

I know I had a severe anxiety phase just before I became progressively hypothyroid with my Hashimoto's thyroiditis. A little better explanation is this; When the thyroid is being damaged by "antibodies", it will cause it to release spurts of too much hormone, as a defense mechanism but as soon as this overdrive mode stops, you drop back down to low levels again.

After a while, the thyroid becomes so damaged, it cannot recover or fight off the autoimmune attack anymore and continues to slip down into progressive hypothyroidism.

I've heard a lot of people's stories about Hashimoto's Disease/hypothyroidism and they related having anxiety attacks when they had too many duties to perform and it overwhelmed them (stress-induced) and other times it just happened to them for no apparent reason (possibly hormone fluctuations). Have you had the "thyroid antibodies" tests (i.e. the TPO and TG antibodies)? You might consider this because it can reveal an autoimmune attack going on, even when thyroid hormone levels are in normal-range.

QUESTION THIRTY-SIX

Any Comments on Thyroid Hormone Therapy and Depression Symptoms?

From my forum reply Re: "Thyroid Hormone Therapy and Depression Symptoms".---

By going to www.thyroid.about.com – website, you then can put in search words; "Depression and Thyroid Disease" in the search-bar that appears at top-page and it will list articles you can click on. I do know there is a belief by some medical experts that depressive thyroid patients need t-3 hormone and not the t-4 only, which is what Synthroid, among other brands contain (needing t-3 may not the case with everyone who has depression). Most, if not all of us who are hypothyroid patients have had depression with our thyroid disorders. Mine completely lifted when my hormone therapy was increased to the correct dose (my TSH needs suppressed to under 1.0) but that's me and who's to say that's right for each person who suffers stubborn depression symptoms. It's worth researching though and I hope the website I suggested helps you with information in regard to this issue. Please also communicate with someone, including posting on thyroid support forums, when you feel down.

In former posts, I speak of my problem with the "antidepressant prescribing craze" but I hope no one thinks I am advocating against SSRI antidepressants themselves. My mother takes Prozac, plus is treated for her underactive thyroid and she does very well.

289

My problem is use of these drugs to treat unrelieved
emotional symptoms when thyroid treatment is not
optimized, when this alone could be the answer for some
people (getting correct thyroid dose levels). If a patient is
not optimized and they are placed on an antidepressant, I
am concerned about their being able to distinguish the
side-effects of the antidepressant, from any unrelieved
thyroid symptoms. I hope that makes sense.

However, some people need help on an immediate basis
and if they know their thyroid hormone medication is at
the correct level, an antidepressant might be just what they
need! No two situations are exactly the same but
GENERALLY, making sure thyroid dose is optimal, is
usually a good idea before accepting a prescribed mood
disorder drug that is usually a long-term or lifelong
treatment.

QUESTION THIRTY-SEVEN

What are Natural and Synthetic T4 and T3 Hormone Therapies?

From my forum reply Re: "Natural and Synthetic T4 and T3 Hormone Therapies" ---

Levothyroxine is just the name for synthetic t-4 hormone replacement medication, which comes in the different brands such as "Synthroid, Levoxyl, Levothroid" etc... They are basically the same thing but some of these are considered generics and many doctors prefer to stick to the major brands, due to generics sometimes being less potent at same dose-levels. I started out on Synthroid but didn't get the expected relief of symptoms, so my Doctor placed me on a combo t-3/t-4 hormone called "Armour", which is a natural version, made from animal thyroid glands – porcine/pigs. Natural brands of thyroid hormone are used for the same thing that these other synthetic types are used for which is; thyroid hormone replacement for hypothyroid patients.

The Doctor who first treated me for hypothyroidism, switched me from the synthetic T-4 only brand I had been taking for about a year, thinking I might have a problem with t-4 to t-3 conversion (a process that occurs naturally in the body but fails to do so in some patients). He switched me, believing I might be a person with the inability to convert t-4 only hormone into the other needed t-3 (more active) hormone, due to my experiencing unrelieved symptoms, while being on the brand hormone I was started on (Synthroid).

Most people don't have a problem with this and looking back I have a feeling mine was more of an "insufficient dose" problem rather than an "impaired conversion" one because my blood TSH level (test used to monitor the therapy) was not suppressed adequately by my dose. Reputable medical sources state that TSH is supposed to be brought down to between 1.0 and 2.0 for proper treatment (TSH elevates with hypothyroidism) and mine was only suppressed down to between 3.0 and 5.0 for at least that first year I was treated.

QUESTION THIRTY-EIGHT

Do you have more Information on Emotional Symptoms and Hypothyroid Treatment?

This article is a forum-response I made Re: "Emotional Symptoms and Hypothyroid Treatment"---

Most of us can relate to most of your symptoms and to the depression which is very common with hypothyroidism. I'm an age-42 man who went from going to the Dr. maybe once every 5 or 6 years, to going very frequently due to sudden worsening of symptoms that actually started years earlier. It was extremely depressing and caused me great anxiety as well, to go from a strong (6ft 215lb), hard working man, to feeling like I could barely walk across a room. I admit now that I actually did become suicidal but by being patient in getting dosage adjustments in treating my hypothyroidism and especially with God's help, I made it through that incredibly tough time. I still have symptom flare-ups and generally have more fatigue at times than I used-to but have improved dramatically!

Please always talk to someone and us too at the forum when you need to. Just put "need help now!" or something to that effect and we'll correspond with you as quickly as we can but let me also encourage you in saying that you will see improvement over time, with thyroid hormone therapy, to treat your hypothyroidism though it seems hard to see right now! You have a Doctor who is trying you on increased dosages and he will keep doing so until you feel better and are in the right range for you to feel better on your hormone dose!

Is so hard to be patient but once you start gaining ground, you will see happiness slowly return and in turn it will bring back your ambition!

Myself and others I've read postings from on this forum, have had the same experience with symptoms being claimed not to be thyroid-related (especially emotional ones), when we know for a fact they are and yes, it is very frustrating. It is also insulting for lingering symptoms to be called psychosomatic (imagined). Many times I actually believe it is simply a matter of what's easier for some Doctors to treat and that's why the emotional diagnosis is used a lot. Of course there are those who would disagree with this and they have that right but I've read so many testimonies of people who went through this and once they had proper treatment for their thyroid disease, the symptoms finally resolved but it usually amounted to finding the right Doctor or in the person finally influencing the Doctor in better treatment options (i.e. dose increases or changing brands).

QUESTION THIRTY-NINE

Is there Risk for Crohn's Disease in thyroid Patients?

This short reply, I made, was to a thyroid patient who was having stomach symptoms, including blood in their stools and symptoms affecting their eyes – Re: "The Risk for Crohn's Disease in thyroid Patients" ---

I've not seen these symptoms mentioned for hypothyroidism before and they do sound serious, needing a Dr's care and investigation.

Most of us have the Autoimmune Type of Hypothyroidism, called Hashimoto's Thyroiditis and as I have researched have found that one autoimmune disease can lead to another, so can co-exist but this would be the only connection I would see.

There is a colon disease called "Crohn's" and I know a man who has this and it too is an autoimmune disease. He had bleeding as you described and also caused him anemia but with treatment, his is in remission and has been for a couple of years now.

Of course I don't know if you have this or even a similar condition but this is an example of a type disease that can cause this and that thyroid patients are at slightly increased risk for developing. This friend also did mention to me that the Crohn's seriously affected his eyes and is also why I mentioned it as a possibility in your case, that your doctor may want to investigate. I hope you find a good physician that can get to the cause and administer the treatment you need soon!

QUESTION FORTY

Can Thyroid Cysts and Hypothyroid Symptoms mean Hashimoto's?

From my forum-reply re: "Thyroid Cysts and Hypothyroid Symptoms can mean Hashimoto's" ---

(My reply was to a forum-poster who described having hypothyroid symptoms and a soft lump on their thyroid gland that could be felt on the outside of their throat.)

The symptoms you described can be thyroid related and related directly to your cyst as well. The cyst may actually be what they call a nodule. Nodules happen in both Hashimoto's Thyroiditis(Hypothyroidism-under active) and in Graves Disease (Hyperthyroidism-overactive). Since though you have spells of both hyperthyroid type symptoms and hypothyroid type symptoms, it could be the Hashimoto's type of thyroid autoimmunity because with Hashimoto's person will go through periods of switching back & forth between both types of symptoms for a while, usually early into the disease, before becoming permanently hypothyroid. It is the thyroid's way of trying to fight off the autoimmune attack, by temporarily increasing its hormone output in attempt to overwhelm the damage and inflammation occurring from antibodies, mistakenly sent from the immune system to attack it.

I would get the "antibodies" blood tests done that can detect autoimmune thyroid disease along with thyroid hormone levels (thyroid panel) because Hashimoto's can exist in people even when hormones are within normal range.

Don't let a Dr. tell you otherwise, it is an established fact confirmed by reputable medical sources. Unfortunately some Dr.s actually don't know this (also a fact). The antibody tests are the "Anti-Thyroglobulin (TG) and Anti-thyroidperoxidase (TPO)" Tests. I would tell the Doctor that you want these done and be firm, not letting him talk you out of these being done. Let us know results if you like, we'll add follow up comments if your antibodies do happen to be elevated.

QUESTION FOURTY-ONE

Any Suggestions Regarding the Thyroid Patient – Doctor Dilemma?

This article is derived from my post Re: "The Thyroid Patient – Doctor Dilemma".---

Many other thyroid patients, posting on forums have attested to experiencing some of the same things with certain Dr.s they have been-to as I have and if it were just a few people reporting these type things, you might say it wasn't a serious problem but I've heard it constantly from a lot of people for many years now. All five Dr.s I first visited for treatment of my thyroid disease, wanted to prescribe me antidepressants (two gave out samples) and except for that first Dr. who prescribed them (tried them about 2-months), I threw them all away if prescribed afterward. My problem-symptoms were joint pain and fatigue but I expressed plainly that if I did have anxiety/depression, it was very mild and a result, rather than a cause of my symptoms. This was all after I started thyroid hormone replacement medication and had gotten well-past the emotional stuff and had only the lingering physical symptoms to deal with, which was due to insufficient hormone dose levels.

After the first two Dr.s prescribed these emotions drugs on several visits to each of them, as I sought help for my fibromyalgia type pain my wife asked to go with me just to see if the next Doctor I changed to, in attempt to get help, would do this as well. She was flabbergasted when he also tried to push these drugs on me within the first 30 secs of that first office visit.

When I changed to a yet another new Doctor again later, she was with me again, when he too immediately reached for the script-pad to prescribe an SSRI Antidepressant. My family, my parents, my friends etc... all knew I did not have emotional issues and in fact I was very optimistic and improved greatly in that area. The drugs were offered simply because I had unrelieved physical symptoms and this apparently was not what these doctors wanted to hear and was an obvious frustration to them.

My TSH the first time I complained of no relief from my thyroid hormone therapy was "4.98" Reference range was 0.5 to 5.0 and after I complained that my dose was too low via search I did on proper TSH levels, my doctor increased my dose to suppress my TSH down to "3.10". This was over nearly two years period of time but each time they would say "YOU'RE IN THE NORMAL RANGE", there's no reason you shouldn't be completely well.

In the mean time, I had all those tests I listed earlier and for all of that time, I SIMPLY NEEDED A DOSAGE INCREASE and my symptoms would have improved. The most reputable medical sources in existence, including the U.S. National Institutes of Health recommend that TSH levels be suppressed down to between "1.0 and 3.0", in treating hypothyroidism with thyroid hormone dosing.

What I discovered was that these less-informed doctors actually believed that ANYTHING within the normal values range (for diagnosing rather than treating hypothyroidism) was acceptable.

They called my remaining symptoms psychosomatic because they did not know about the importance of optimizing treatment (dose-titration) and it was easier for them to prescribe an SSRI antidepressant, rather than adjusting my dose to accomplish this. I spent a ton of unnecessary money for tests to diagnose other possible causes of my symptoms, when adequate dosing was what I was lacking and in need of.

Some people suggest that this type of scenario that is happening to patients is due to over-booking of Office Visits and high Medical Liability Insurance Costs for Doctors. I'm sure these are two of the major reasons but are still a terrible thing to be experienced by patients regardless of these factors. It is people like us who are free to express our grievances that can make a difference for others who are suffering these type things and I hope reform of these problems will someday take place but it won't happen any time soon if the problem is not recognized by those who have the authority to help it change for the better.

QUESTION FOURTY-TWO

Is there a way to distinguish between Good Thyroid Doctors versus Bad Ones?

From my post Re: "Good Thyroid Doctors Versus Bad Ones". ---

My Mother has a Dr. that is absolutely sensational! He is not cold and indifferent but actually listens to the patient without patronizing them. I have tried to get in with him several times, over several years but he is booked-up and there is a long waiting list. Other experiences I've had with past Dr.s were pathetic and I don't know any other way to express a bad experience other than to tell it "the way it was". To not warn people about the "obvious things" that are happening, such as people being treated with antidepressants, when the root cause is untreated thyroid disease or other serious health disorder, would be just as much a disservice to them as it would be to not give them the good information in regard to qualified thyroid doctors who are out there. AND, if we suggest something to possibly research and look into as fellow-patients through forums, it might be more of a process of elimination, than the actual answer but can still be helpful on many different levels!

The people posting on patient support forums KNOW we are fellow patients and we try to give as many views as we can without getting too outrageous. In my opinion, I would rather have several possibilities to research-out than only one "iffy one" suggested by a doctor who has not taken time to thoroughly evaluate my case.

301

I had Doctors suggest possibilities for my symptoms in my case, including Rheumatoid Arthritis (ruled-out by RA Factor test), Gout (ruled-out by Uric Acid Test), Low-Testosterone (ruled by blood and saliva testing), Diabetes (ruled-out by glucose-average 90 day test – A1C), Addison's Disease (ruled-out by ACTH Stim. Test), Allergies (ruled-out by blood-allergens test), etc.... This was AFTER being on thyroid medication for over two years but through research on my own, I found that I was not in the optimal TSH range to feel better from my thyroid hormone therapy, so increased my dosage through a new Doctor and "Presto!" I got much better!

It was other thyroid patients who warned me about the possibility of "under treatment" and that it was a fairly common problem but 2-Doctors actually laughed at me when I suggested under treatment and they basically said "leave the treatment to us". How wonderful it would have been if I could have actually done that and been properly diagnosed and treated earlier and saved all that money! HINDSIGHT is an advantage and is exactly what patients who've been through this type thing have on their side, that they can warn others patients about! To not share the pitfalls along with the positives is like giving only half an answer to a question of great importance. Thank God for the excellent Dr.s who are out there! They are to be praised! But, patients desperately need to recognize inferior treatment when it does happen, so that they can exercise their right to a second opinion.

QUESTION FOURTY-THREE

Is Thyroid Patient Education and Proactiveness Important?

This article is derived from my post Re: "Thyroid Patient Education and Proactiveness".---

I just recently found information about hot and cold nodules (thyroid tumors) and I believe a "hot" one, causes the thyroid to continually release hormone and causes hyperthyroidism such as what Graves' disease people have (autoimmune hyperthyroidism – overactive).

A nodule, may cause transient hyperthyroidism for a while, like Hashimoto's thyroiditis people have (autoimmune hypothyroidism – under active, preceded by temporary hyperthyroidism) when the thyroid is fizzling out but then becomes a "cold nodule" and no longer elevates hormone production from the gland.

Since you've had hypothyroid readings and high antibodies (per your post), yours is almost certainly the Hashimoto's kind of thyroid autoimmunity and is also why the Doctor didn't see a need in further scanning your gland (radioactive imaging) at this point.

There is a site created by a Hashimoto's-Man called "HateShopping" (not certain if the site is still up or if it is under a new domain-name) and if you are able to go there, click on his article titled "WHY YOU ARE NOT CRAZY".

He has other very good ones too but in this one he relates how Dr.s misdiagnosed him as "Bi-Polar, Schizophrenic" etc..., in other words, the old "psychosomatic" catch-all diagnoses, rather than blood testing him for possible diseases, including thyroid – the one he was eventually diagnosed with. He also relates on the site, having had hyperthyroid symptoms with his Hashimoto's, with rapid heart beat and elevated blood pressure. He too knocks negative experiences he's had with Dr.s but also mentions there are many out there who are trustworthy.

YES, I admit I've been very passionate in trying to inform others about the importance of patient-proactiveness and self-education because of mine, my wife's, my mother's, my Uncle's etc.... - experiences in not getting diagnosed properly, without the tremendous added expense of changing Dr.s, wrong tests being ordered, etc.... This is why I SO APPRECIATE thyroid patient advocates like Mary Shomon who by the way, has a book called "Living Well With Hypothyroidism", and I highly recommend it and her other book "Living Well With Autoimmune Disease". NO, she's not a Doctor but here are examples of Dr.s who endorsed her books; Stephen Langer MD, Marie Savard MD, Larian Gillespie MD, Carol Roberts MD, David Brownstien MD,etc... What do you know – a thyroid patient with experience and knowledge!

Also: Dr. Lowe is Director of Research for the "Fibromyalgia Research Foundation" and has a "B.A., M.A., B.S., AND a doctorate in Chiropractic. His education exceeds that needed to be a Chiropractic Dr. and thankfully research like the foundation he is involved in, is ongoing for fibromyalgia and thyroid patients.

304

His research agrees with that by many other Dr.s and researchers like "Mary Shomon", who is not a Dr. but is recognized by the medical community as one of the leading authorities on thyroid disease. She has a series of books on the subject, endorsed by many Dr.s. I personally, will take good information from any source I can get it and I always confirm it by my own research of other sources that compare with it.

QUESTION FOURTY-FOUR

Is Diagnosing and Monitoring Thyroid Disease by Blood the Best Way?

From my post Re: "Diagnosing and Monitoring Thyroid Disease by Blood".---

Doctors after all these years of advancement in thyroid disease diagnosis and treatments, should know that people with autoimmune thyroid diseases (Both Hashimoto's thyroiditis & Graves' disease), can have full blown symptoms even when hormone lab-ranges are still within normal range. Many reputable medical sites I read stated that "high antibody levels" prevent thyroid hormones from binding to receptor sites (process of taking them into the cells of the body to regulate metabolism), even when hormone levels are adequate, causing hypothyroidism symptoms. They especially should know that the TSH test alone will miss a lot of borderline cases of developing thyroid disease as well – especially those that are developing due to antibodies attacking the thyroid gland (autoimmunity).

That would be right at almost 4-weeks (per your post) for a new thyroid hormone dose to take effect and this is supposed to be long enough for it to change your lab ranges as much as it's going to but some doctors allow for 6 to 8 weeks to make certain. When I go for retesting of my thyroid hormone levels, to monitor my therapy, I will usually only skip the dose for that morning until the blood is drawn, then take it afterward.

I do this because thyroid hormone has at least a few hours half life (the natural type/brands like Armour) and the synthetic (like Synthroid) has a half life of several days, so should still be built up in your system and not cause much problem by delaying a dose on one day. It is my opinion however, and Dr.s may actually disagree with this, that taking a thyroid hormone dose the same morning, just before blood is drawn for a retest, may show inaccurately/falsely high medication levels because it hasn't been absorbed into the cells of the body yet and is still mostly in the blood stream. The makers of Armour actually suggest delaying your dose on the morning of a blood draw.

QUESTION FOURTY-FIVE

What are the Far-Reaching Effects of Thyroid Antibodies?

This article is from my forum post Re: "The Far-Reaching Effects of Thyroid Antibodies".---

I've researched about "Sub-Acute Thyroiditis" but understood it to be temporary as you stated and I don't believe it causes the elevated antibodies you have, as stated on your post. I could be wrong about that, so you might try a search on it using that name but I'm fairly certain it doesn't typically cause thyroid antibodies to develop or at least not to significant (flagged high) levels.

I have Hashimoto's Hypothyroidism but I didn't have an antibodies test for two years, I only new my thyroid was low functioning. I finally had an antibodies test, May this year (2005) and my TOP ABs were "84" (normal being <35) and my TG ABs were "537" (normal being <40). My Doctor indicated that high antibody levels can cause symptoms even when thyroid hormone levels are at normal-range and I researched this fact and found lots of confirming information on it.

I also found studies in which many Dr.s believe fibromyalgia & Chronic Fatigue Syndrome are often thyroid-related. I hope yours is the temporary type of thyroiditis but with those antibody levels, it looks like Hashimoto's thyroiditis – the permanent type that eventually results in progressive hypothyroidism.

Thyroid patient Advocate - Mary Shomon is a Hashimoto's sufferer and recognized as one of the nations top authorities on the subject. She did a survey (Quality of Life Survey of Thyroid Patients) in 2003 and results have just recently been released. A group of 860 Hypo/Hashi people, with TSH levels in optimal range, reported still having symptoms as follows; 789 (92%) still had fatigue/exhaustion despite treatment. Over 500 still had weight gain/unable to lose. 437 still had joint/muscle pain etc.......... It is a very revealing survey in regard to this disease and the effectiveness of treatment for it. My belief is that antibody levels cause the lingering symptoms in some patients, so we need diet exercise and all around better taking care of ourselves to help improve them, in addition to our thyroid hormone replacement therapy.

QUESTION FOURTY-SIX

Any Ideas Regarding Highly Elevated Thyroid Antibodies and Steroid Treatment?

From my forum post regarding "Highly Elevated Thyroid Antibodies and Steroid Treatment".---

The ATHYP means Anti-Thyro-Peroxidase Antibodies test (also sometime abbreviated "TPO") and the ATHYG means Anti-Thyro-Globulin Antibodies test (also sometimes abbreviated "TG"). If your TPO ABs were elevated but not the TG ones, this still means autoimmune thyroid disease most likely because some people only have one or the other elevated and some have both elevated.

The corticosteroid treatment you mention is sometimes given short-term to reduce inflammation in patients who appear to have a high level of it. It is a hydrocortisone steroid, like "Prednisone", which a Dr. gave me short-term, in my own case, when he saw I had high antibody readings of both types. These corticosteroids are given for many inflammatory diseases, sometimes short term and sometimes long term (such as for rheumatoid arthritis, Addison's Disease etc…) As was my case, doctors may give steroid treatment to patients, if they feel they are at risk for Hashimoto's encephalitis is (HE), which is a severe and sometimes life-threatening neurological response to elevated thyroid antibodies.

My TPO Antibodies were "84" (range at the lab was <35) and my TG Antibodies were "537" (Range at the lab was <45).

In my case, the thyroglobulins were much higher than the peroxidase ones, although they were considerably above normal too. It's strange that labs vary on their normal ranges and sometimes, it's a matter of where they place the decimal point and whether they add one or not. Your test had a normal range on the TPO of <2, but I've seen ones that had "0-74" as the normal range (not sure why they vary from lab to lab). Yours would still be flagged "high" even at this higher normal range.

Hypothyroid patients even without HE, sometimes have neurological symptoms and I think Dr.s are now learning this to be more common than originally thought. There was a time I would wake up in the night, early into my own disease, feeling like I was having a little seizure and I would feel a strange pain on one side of my tongue, at the same time. It was a weird sensation but I felt sure it was the hypothyroidism, rather than hints of HE because they also list "tingling & numbness in hands, arms, feet & legs" as a hypothyroid symptom on some medical sources.

QUESTION FOURTY-SEVEN

Any Suggestions for Dealing with Hashimoto's Disease and Hypothyroidism?

The following is derived from my forum post regarding "Dealing with Hashimoto's Disease and Hypothyroidism".---

I would say that your TSH of "8.87" is considerably elevated, but it is hard to give more specific feedback without knowing the ranges on the test. These are found on your results and look something like this - "Range: 0.4 to 4.0". I have read numerous articles that have listed soy (per your mention of soy in your diet) as a contributing factor to thyroid problems.

Testing high for thyroid antibodies probably means you have Hashimotos Disease, which is a progressive autoimmune thyroiditis that over time will make your thyroid fail to function. You may have only noticed the fatigue symptom so far – as you related, but you've probably had some symptoms you disregarded as being something like stress, aging or working to hard, just like the fatigue you mention as being "vague". Hashimoto's disease can make your symptoms manifest as either hypothyroid (under active) or hyperthyroid (overactive) in its early stages but always becomes a progressive hypothyroid disease, eventually.

Some of my own symptoms as a Hashimoto's – hypothyroid patient have been dry skin, heart flutters, fatigue, mind fog, forgetful, anxiety, etc...

My best advice at this point is to stop the soy and start your prescribed hormone replacement meds. You may go through some strange feelings after starting the medication (adjustment symptoms) like heart flutters, maybe even some hair loss, but by continuing to take them; you will feel better over time. I also found information, stating that soy can have negative affect on hypothyroid patients, being a "goitrogen food" (potentially lowers thyroid hormones). Your antibodies are highly elevated, per your posted results. Your TSH @ 8.87 indicates your thyroid is already struggling to keep up with your body's hormone needs. Your T-4 is almost borderline-low, further proof your hormone levels are dropping from the autoimmune attack on your thyroid gland. Even your Thyroglobulin Antibodies (TG) are elevated but not near as much as the other ones (TPO –antithyroidperoxidase).

It sounds like your Dr. has positively diagnosed you as having Hashimoto's. His advice to you sounds good about needing dosage adjustments due to the antibodies being elevated because they will cause more damage to your thyroid over time. I've heard some sources on websites say that the antibodies also attack your replacement hormone as it enters your body but I'm not sure there is any medically confirmed proof of that. Weight gain can definitely happen despite treatment and is hard for me to lose weight too. I'm 6ft., 215lb but can't seem to reduce from this but will fluctuate up to 220 instead. I almost quit eating at one time out of frustration (not a good idea) and still didn't lose weight (STRANGE). I don't mind being big, since I'm a man but wanted more energy and any extra pounds does not help me in this area, so I continue to work on personal weight loss.

QUESTION FOURTY-EIGHT

Is Thyroid Autoimmunity – a Major Factor in Symptoms?

This article is from a post I made in regard to "Thyroid Autoimmunity – a Major Factor in Symptoms".---

I would like to say that I like many thyroid patients, went through 5 Doctors before receiving a proper diagnosis. I was diagnosed with Generalized Anxiety Disorder, depression, psycho-somatic symptoms etc..... and It was due to my being given the run-around that I finally insisted on diagnostic blood tests and the diagnosis of my thyroid disease (Hashimoto's-hypothyroidism) was properly made. What's funny is that I suggested "thyroid disorder" to that very first Dr. I visited with my symptoms because I knew beyond-doubt that my condition had a medical/physical cause, with emotional symptoms being only one aspect of it.

There was a survey done by Thyroid Patient Advocate - Mary Shomon in 2003 of 1000 thyroid patients. I realize she is literally shunned by some in the Medical Community but is praised by just as many reputable people practicing in the Medical field. In this survey, which was the first and largest of its kind, over HALF of patients on thyroid replacement hormone therapy for hypothyroidism and with TSH ranges at optimal range, still had lingering symptoms such as joint pain, serious fatigue, depression etc...

314

This tells me, it is neither the doctors nor the patients in many cases but is often the "autoimmune component" of thyroid disease itself that causes or contributes-to symptoms and not whether the thyroid hormones are treated to get them into the optimal range or not.

If symptoms that continue, even while on treatment, are so rare in treated thyroid patients, why would a survey of this sort have these type results and why are SO MANY online patients with autoimmune thyroid disease, seemingly in the very same boat in regard to unsatisfactory symptom relief? Are there this many psycho-somatic people? No, but rather there are many patients who suffer from the effects of an autoimmune process that is affecting their body, causing inflammation and alterations in their immune system function. In my personal but firm opinion, this is the most important factor contributing to unsatisfactory results in some treated hypothyroid patients and there are medical research studies that point to this fact as well.

315

QUESTION FOURTY-NINE

Can Goiters occur with Hashimoto's Thyroiditis?

This article is derived from my forum post on the subject of "Goiters that can occur with Hashimoto's Thyroiditis".

Yes, it does sound like Hashimoto's disease (description of thyroid problem given by a forum-poster) although there is a type of "thyroiditis", called Painful Thyroiditis - a temporary condition that clears up after a while (4 to 6 weeks). I'm not saying yours will hurt permanently but a lot of Hashi's people have pain in their thyroid glands that comes and goes. Other patients experience pain temporary pain in their glands once and after that, the pain never returns. Non-painful goiters and mildly painful goiters are fairly common with Hashimoto's thyroiditis. Some people have large swelling and never any pain, who knows for sure why it manifests differently among patients. Other Hashi's patients never experience a significant goiter and some only develop small nodules and only mild goiters (me included).

If you've been diagnosed hypothyroidism, it is almost certainly caused by lifetime thyroiditis (it's the most common cause in industrialized countries) and if you tested positive for antibodies, this helps confirm that the hypothyroidism is caused by the autoimmune Hashimoto's disease. You might do an online search on "Goiters Caused by Hashimoto's" and this will probably yield a lot of information.

If you see cancerous nodules mentioned, don't let that scare you because it is extremely rare and if you know you have Hashi's, you know that's the cause of your nodules. I've had slight dull aches in my thyroid gland from time to time.

I may be sticking my neck out a little now but when I had a problem in the past getting a Dr. to order me an antibodies with my having recurrent symptoms and dosage problems with my thyroid replacement medication, I found websites that set up blood testing/no with Dr. visit required. They send results directly to you and you simply have your blood drawn at one of their network of locations (usually doctor's offices that participate). There are several of these firms out there that offer the blood testing, which is completed by reputable labs, such as Quest or LabCorp. The one I used was www.healthcheckusa.com (networking through LabCorp) and the tests were also less expensive than I was able to get through my doctor's office or local hospital. They tell you the closest location you can have blood drawn at (within miles of you) and you get blood drawn there - no office visit.

If you have a Doc that refuses you a test, I would consider a firm like the one I describe above. There are many now out there, which helps people to have blood tests done that they find difficulty getting ordered through their doctors for whatever reasons.

QUESTION FIFTY

Any Comments on Adrenal Fatigue and Thyroid Hormone Therapy?

This is a forum post I made in 2005, regarding my experience with "Adrenal Fatigue and Thyroid Hormone Therapy".---

Back when I first was diagnosed with hypothyroidism, I didn't get the expected symptom relief from my thyroid hormone replacement therapy and research I did on this problem and the potential causes of it, mentioned that LOW adrenal hormones (low cortisol) could worsen symptoms of adrenal insufficiency if you start thyroid hormone medication but do not first correct the hypo-cortisolism. As far as HIGH cortisol, there is probably an effect there as well because your thyroid and adrenal hormones interact and some medical sources even call it the "Thyroid-Adrenal-Axis". Clinically low cortisol is called "Addison's Disease" and high cortisol is called "Cushing's Disease" (use these terms to search these conditions online).

I did several home adrenal hormone saliva tests (four over a year period) that showed I had consistently low cortisol levels but probably not severe enough to be called Addison's disease and more probably a sub clinical but significant type of "adrenal Fatigue" or adrenal exhaustion. None of my Dr.s took it seriously, so to this day I still have a degree of it that can come in flares and cause me concerning symptoms, including a lowered tolerance for stress (stressors).

I had the 24-hour urine cortisol measure done as well, which also revealed that my level of the hormone was low.

The range for adult males age 18 and over was <119 and my result was "10.7". Even my doctor at the time admitted my level was one of the lowest he had ever seen on this test. Despite this fact, I am required to treat the adrenal fatigue myself with safe, natural adrenal boosting supplements because doctors do not recognize low adrenal function unless it is severe enough to require cortisol replacement therapy (cortical steroid drugs).

QUESTION FIFTY-ONE

Is Getting Leveled-out on Thyroid Hormone Replacement Difficult?

This article is derived from my forum post regarding "Getting Leveled-out on Thyroid Hormone Replacement".---

With your TSH going from 0.15 to 7.63, this definitely looks like Hashimoto's Disease (autoimmune hypothyroidism) because you are going from a hyperthyroid to a hypothyroid reading on blood labs, within a short space of time. If I understand correctly, Graves Disease causes a constant hyperthyroid state, so much so, that it endangers some people with severe cases of having uncontrollable hypertension and tachycardia (rapid heart rate) and they end up having to remove or destroy their thyroid gland, then place them on thyroid replacement hormone. Yours sure sounds like the often present swings Hashimoto's patients have. I too have had intermittent hyperthyroid times but mine declined into hypothyroidism fairly shortly after a few weeks of hyperthyroid symptoms (Hashitoxicosis) and then stayed hypothyroid from that time on. I now take 150mg of Armour Thyroid brand hormone medication for my case.

Levoxyl is the name for synthetic T-4 (often prescribed via the Synthroid brand) and Dr.s usually prescribe it more often than the natural forms, the most well known natural type being Armour as I referred-to earlier, which is a combination of both T-3 & T-4. I was actually first started on Synthroid and switched to Armour by a doctor who thought the brand might be superior in my case.

The problem in SOME PEOPLE is that their system won't naturally convert the T-4 only hormone, into the other needed "T-3" hormone. They call this an "impaired hormone conversion problem". The T-3 is actually the more "active" form of thyroid hormone. Some people do just fine on the synthetic T-4 (my own mother does for example).

On the other hand some people don't tolerate the natural Armour type medication because it causes them spells of hyperthyroid type symptoms (T3 sensitivity) but I've personally never had that problem. Another thing people aren't aware of (me included until I found out) is that when you take thyroid medication, your own thyroid cuts back on it's own production of hormone (atrophy of the gland). This means if you are not taking "full replacement dosage", for a while you will just break-even and not experience immediate improvement in low thyroid symptoms. That's why Dr.s have you re-test several times especially at the beginning of administering a new dose, until it is in the right range via blood retesting. That's why some people (I was one of them) feel no difference at all for a while because you simply break even until you get the right amount in you that is adequate to restore metabolism in the body.

It's too bad there are so many of these crazy issues that can affect our treatment but all we can do, is the best we can!

QUESTION FIFTY-TWO

Should I be Firm in Requesting Thyroid Blood Testing?

My reply on a forum Re: "Being Firm in Requesting Thyroid Blood Testing".---

All the symptoms you describe sound like classic hypothyroid symptoms; in fact it is almost like reading a list from a medical site! The cysts you refer-to are probably "nodules" (small benign tumors in the gland) but your Dr. will need to determine for sure.

Nodules and goiters (thyroid enlargement & bumps), are common with autoimmune thyroid disease, which is the most common cause of hypothyroidism (low thyroid function). It is also called Hashimoto's Thyroiditis.

Request (firmly) that your Dr. to order a thyroid panel with "thyroid antibodies" tests along with it. I say to be firm in requesting these because he is working for you, not the other way around and your health is an important possession, worthy of through evaluation. I'm not telling you to be rude but do be firm because you are your own advocate in getting proper care.

YES, Dr.s will sometimes act arrogant towards patients and think it is ridiculous for them to suggest a test etc... but if one is too reluctant to see the importance of through evaluation, it may be time for a new Dr..

It is your body and you have rights, as a patient to protect your life and ability to continue with your livelihood and support of your family.

322

Also make sure they give you photo-copies of all lab results because YOU PAY FOR THEM and they are obliged by "HIPPA law" to provide them upon your request (may require signing a release). This way, it will help you in case you want to research the results online or share them with others, like us of fellow-patient forums.

I am a Hashimoto's – hypothyroidism patient, as are many on this forum.

QUESTION FIFTY-THREE

Is there a Relationship of TSH and Thyroid Antibodies to Hypothyroid Symptoms?

My forum comment Re: "Relationship of TSH and Thyroid Antibodies to Hypothyroid Symptoms".---

First, that TSH reading (3.9) is actually high for a hypothyroid patient on thyroid replacement medication. Every reputable site I have ever looked at to see what recommendations were for TSH levels in patients on replacement hormone medication said it should be between 1.0 to 2.0 but they also say that some patients only have relief of symptoms when theirs is less than 1.0. You can actually get down to 0.35 and not yet be in hyperthyroidism territory. I've had mine down to 0.45 and had no hyper type symptoms at all, in fact I still had some hypothyroid symptoms until mine was lowered/suppressed even more with an increased dose (my T4 and T3 would remain in normal range).

The "American Association of Clinical Endocrinologists" came out with NEW GUIDELINES for TSH levels in 2002 and most labs have not re-adjusted their ranges as yet. This organization which is the most reliable source for endocrinology standards (thyroid is in this category), issued the new guidelines for TSH as being "0.3 to 3.0" and stated that anyone with a TSH of 3.0 is suspect for hypothyroidism. With yours being 3.9, you could easily still be hypothyroid! If you'll do a search and put in key words "New TSH standards", you'll find these new guidelines.

Your Microsomal antibodies also sound very high but I'm not familiar with that name and is likely the same as the TPO antibodies (antithyroidperoxidase). Usually the other ones they check are called the Anti-Thyroglobulin – abbreviated "TG" (which you noted was normal) and the TPO ones. Did the microsomal one have a reference range? I can almost guarantee that microsomal level/result you posted (in the 100s) is HIGH! But, I would like to see the normal values range. Usually a range will look like this: "<70" or something to that effect, meaning your antibodies should be that number or less. That's the same range my lab had on the antithyroidperoxidase one, so that reading you reported is very high in comparison to that type of range! Some people with Hashimoto's thyroiditis have only one or the other that's high (positive) and some have both of them high but it's my understanding that the TPO one is even more important than the TG one.

I don't know a great deal about the ANA (anti-nuclear antibodies) test, as it relates to thyroid disease except that mine was negative when I had it tested. Antibodies are suppose to go down over time with thyroid hormone medication but some medical sites I have read/searched, said that it can take years for this to occur. I feel high antibodies can cause symptoms as much as low hormone levels can and there are medical studies confirming this fact.

QUESTION FIFTY-FOUR

Can Thyroid Antibodies Cause Chronic Hives?

My forum post regarding "Thyroid Antibodies can Cause Chronic Hives".---

You don't see hives mentioned on very many medical sites but high level (positive) thyroid antibodies can cause them. The reason I searched about this is because I came down with severe hives just before being diagnosed with Hashimoto's Disease but did not make the connection until two years later, when I found mention of it happening with Hashimoto's thyroiditis, on medical research sources.

I had NEVER had hives before and not since being treated for hypothyroidism but they are always an immune system reaction (i.e. from allergies or antibodies) or in response to tremendous stress (traumatic or chronic). I agree that they should run thyroid panel blood tests for your son, due to his unexplainable hives - also called "chronic uticaria" and keep blood testing any areas of suspicion until an answer is found for what is causing them. My "Eos"(eosinophils) were also flagged "high" when blood testing was ordered to find my Hashimoto's/hypothyroidism thyroid disorder, which indicated an allergy, which may have also contributed to mine.

QUESTION FIFTY-FIVE

Are there any Basic Questions New Thyroid Patients should ask Doctors?

My forum post Re: "Basic Questions New Thyroid Patients should Ask Doctors".---

Your diagnosis of hypothyroidism is due to your TSH being elevated and as far as the T-4 level, I would need to see the range the lab used as a reference. Your TSH though is definitely elevated above normal because most labs have a range on it of about 0.5 to 5.0. The reason TSH elevates is because your thyroid is under active and TSH (Thyroid Stimulating Hormone), is trying to get your low functioning thyroid to produce more hormone, as your levels have begun to drop. Did they check your thyroid antibody levels? This would be the Anti-Thyroglobulin and Anti-Thyroperoxidase Antibodies.

These two tests are to see if autoimmune disease of the thyroid is causing the hypothyroidism. There are other causes, so this test would be helpful if you have not already been ordered these. Have they or are they going to place you on thyroid hormone replacement medication? Have they mentioned you having a goiter or nodule (tumor in your gland)? These are questions you might ask your doctor if he has not already gone over these issues with you. Also, a really good information source is the thyroid.about.com website (by: Mary Shomon) but you'll get good research info by simply going to a search engine and putting in key words like "hypothyroidism,hashimoto's thyroiditis, thyroid disorders" etc...

Also make sure you get your own copies of every test you have done. You pay for them and it's your right by law to obtain them. This way, it will help you with research you do and questions you ask of other patients like us at this forum. If you have your lab report, post for us all the readings on it, including the reference ranges and we might be able to comment more.

QUESTION FIFTY-SIX

When are Antidepressants needed by Treated Thyroid Patients?

From my forum post Re: "When Antidepressants are Needed by Treated Thyroid Patients".---

The people on this forum always give such good advice! I too am a Hashimoto's/Hypothyroidism sufferer and Dr.s were constantly trying to put me on antidepressants, in fact the first Dr. I visited suggested them and I went ahead and took them for a few months then had to stop them slowly/gradually because my untreated thyroid disease worsened!

I then realized even when I did finally get tested for thyroid disease and was placed on medication/treatment for it, that it would be hard to distinguish the side effects of an antidepressant from unrelieved thyroid symptoms, had I continued them.

Please don't take this as a recommendation to stop your antidepressant; this should NEVER be done apart from doctor-supervision. If you are getting thyroid treatment simultaneously with the antidepressant, this might work for you, if both are needed.

I would however, read thoroughly, the drug-insert that came with the antidepressant or go online and search "side effects of (your drugs name)". Also, never stop taking an antidepressant suddenly. These have to be weaned off of, very gradually and with professional medical supervision.

ALSO, you can have both hyperthyroid and hypothyroid symptoms at the same time. In fact there is an article on this by same title "Can I Be Hypothyroid and Hyperthyroid at The Same Time?" (By: MaryShomon), just go to a search engine and put these search-words in and I bet it'll pop up and be very informative in regard to your case of having symptoms of both.

Lastly, have they tested your thyroid antibody levels? If not, you might request this.

QUESTION FIFTY-SEVEN

Are Mood Disorders Common with Thyroid Disease?

My forum post Re: "Mood Disorders are Common with Thyroid Disease".---

I hope you finally get an attentive, compassionate Dr. this time. Most of us have been through a few that weren't very caring. You never know when a new more specialized Dr. might have much better revelations for you. The "Free T-3 and Free T-4" I have heard are the best thyroid hormones to get tested, as opposed to just T-3 and T-4, which are also called by names such as "Total T-4, Thyroxin", etc... The ones with "Free" in front of them, measure the free, unbound hormone levels, which they say are the best to get tested for superior accuracy.

If they try to indicate that you're a mental case, set them straight! Low mood and anxiety commonly co-exist with thyroid disorders and they should know this but sometimes they try to convince patients that the symptoms are psycho-somatic (emotionally caused) but research I've done states that only about 20% of Major Depression sufferers have severe fatigue and serious joint pain is not as common with emotional problems as they would like us to think (body aches are usually vague with mood disorders).

I asked several people with severe depression but no thyroid disease, if they had joint aches with their mood disorder and they didn't even know what I was talking about.

331

My belief is that so many Dr.s, for so many years have treated medical conditions like thyroid with antidepressants (which won't work, unless the disease is treated too), that they really do believe joint swelling, chronic fatigue etc... are all emotional manifestations. I hope this trend will someday stop, so that needed diagnoses and treatments can be received by more people needing them!

332

QUESTION FIFTY-EIGHT

What is the Purpose of Thyroid Antibody Testing?

A FORUM POST I MADE Re: "The Purpose of Thyroid Antibody Testing".---

The thyroid antibodies test is to see if your hypothyroidism is caused by autoimmune disease (Hashimoto's). Autoimmune disease occurs when your body produces antibodies against an organ/gland, as if it is an intruder. Normally antibodies attack true invaders such as viruses and germs etc... but for some reason the body recognizes part of itself as an invader.

Dr.s don't yet know the reason this happens but in the case of the thyroid, it causes tissue destruction that is irreversible, which results in reduced ability for it to produce adequate hormone levels (hypothyroidism).

Don't let this scare you because it is the most common cause of hypothyroidism in industrialized countries. This is the kind I have. My Anti-Thyroglobulins ABs were "537" (normal range was <35) and my Anti-Thyroperoxidase ABs were "84" (normal being <40), so elevated levels of these are how they determine if you have Hashimoto's thyroiditis (name after the Dr. who discovered it in 1912).

Another reason they check for thyroid antibodies is because autoimmune diseases many times run together, in fact Hashimoto's and Autoimmune Adrenal Insufficiency (Addison's Disease) Co-Exist fairly often.

333

The Dr. probably wants to see if you could possibly have "Schmidt's Syndrome" (Hypothyroid & Addison's combined) or a polyglandular disease of another kind. I hope you don't have one of these combination disorders but there are treatments for them that keep people running normal by replacing any needed hormones that are low. For low thyroid, they give you thyroid hormone replacement and for low adrenal they usually give you hydrocortisone and/or fludrocortisone.

QUESTION FIFTY-NINE

Any Advice Regarding Hypothyroid Treatment and Adrenal Fatigue?

From my forum post Re: "Hypothyroid Treatment and Adrenal Fatigue".---

It's seems I have something in common with so many people on this forum. I too felt I had adrenal insufficiency along with my Hashimoto's/Hypothyroidism because I had worsened hypothyroid symptoms after starting my thyroid hormone replacement medication and I had read this can happen if you have a degree of low-adrenal function and you don't treat it before starting thyroid medication. So, I started out by doing home saliva-tests offered by Great Smokey Mountain Diagnostic Labs, Inc., who market cortisol/DHEA adrenal hormone tests under the name "BodyBalance StressChek". The first one I had done showed low-normal cortisol, so I did a second one a few months later and it showed clinically low levels of cortisol (the major stress/adrenal hormone).

I took these labs to my Dr. and had me do an ACTH Stimulation test (designed to detect full-blown adrenal insufficiency). I passed the test, so he said it wasn't "Addison's Disease" (true adrenal gland disease) however, there are secondary forms of adrenal insufficiency that cause low cortisol levels, which he seemed to not know about. Anyway, I also did a 24-hour urinary cortisol test which also came out very low (range for adult males was <119, mine was "10.7"). I truly believe my cortisol levels dropped even further when I started my thyroid medication.

I can guarantee that your better informed Dr. is testing you because of concern your adrenal insufficiency might be worsened if not treated along with your hypothyroidism, if it does happen to be low. Some medical sites state that Hashimoto's and adrenal insufficiency often co-exist, due to the autoimmune process that can be common with both. They actually have a name for it "Schmidt's Disease" and if you have several low functioning glands, including pancreas (diabetes) and pernicious anemia, they call it "Polyglandular Autoimmune Disease II". I hope they find yours to only be a mild secondary adrenal insufficiency. Your Dr. is wise in checking for this. Most Dr.s don't test for comorbid adrenal dysfunction even though it is even recommended in the Physicians Desk Reference, that adrenal hormones need checked BEFORE thyroid hormone is administered in a patient. A lot of Dr.s have no idea about these things, which is a bit scary but it sounds like you have a good one who has your interests at heart!

One more thing to keep in mind is that LOW-normal thyroid hormones and HIGH-normal TSH readings are sometimes not really normal especially if you have elevated (positive) thyroid antibodies levels. Example: TSH can be in a range of 0.5 to 5.0 but if your result is "4.9" it is well worth further observation. Example: Free T-3 range 2.4 to 4.5 if yours is "2.5" it is worth further observation. When I was diagnosed hypothyroid, my TSH was "8.3" but all other hormones were in low-normal. I later found out that my thyroid antibodies were highly elevated and was why I had full-blown symptoms. I did also have a low T-3 Uptake but they still called it "sub-Clinical" hypothyroidism. Hormones can fluctuate during the autoimmune attack with Hashimoto's thyroiditis (type I have).

QUESTION SIXTY
When is it Important to Determine the Cause of Hypothyroidism?

From my forum post Re: "Determining the Cause of Hypothyroidism".---

That is for sure an elevated TSH level (10.0 and above) because most labs have a range of about 0.5 to 5.0. My TSH at the time I was diagnosed hypothyroid was "8.3" and I also had a T-3 Uptake flagged "low". If they didn't do more tests than this (TSH only), I'm willing to bet they probably will at some point. Make sure you tell them you want the thyroid antibodies panel and don't let them talk you out of it! This test will tell you if the hypothyroidism is due to autoimmune disease or if negative, that it's possibly another reason.

My antibodies were as follows on mine:

Anti-thyroglobulin "537" (normal being <40)

Anti-thyroperoxidase "84" (normal being <35).

Dr.s are not always as knowledgeable about thyroid disorders as you might think and will tell you it doesn't matter what's causing the hypothyroidism however, it does matter because Hashimoto'sThyroiditis is an autoimmune disease and the most common cause of hypothyroidism in industrialized countries. Autoimmune Disease needs close monitoring because you are susceptible to other autoimmune diseases when one is present.

It can also cause goiter (thyroid enlargement) and nodules (thyroid gland tumors) but these are usually easily manageable with thyroid hormone replacement medication which also helps control your hypo symptoms. Let us know about future labs for more comments when we are able. You might also do some search engine research. Just put in key words like "hypothyroidism, Hashimoto's Disease", etc... There is also an informative sight at www.thyroid.about.com published by Thyroid Patient Advocate – Mary Shomon.

QUESTION SIXTY-ONE

Can one have both Hypothyroid and Hyperthyroid Symptoms?

From my forum post Re: "Having both Hypothyroid and Hyperthyroid Symptoms".---

Your heart palpitations and lack of weight gain sounds more in the hyperthyroidism category, however, they most likely came to the hypothyroidism conclusion because of lab results. Did you have blood tests? If so, do you know what your results and the reference ranges were? If they did not provide you a copy of your lab work, I would request one because you pay for these and should be given a copy of all labs done. If you can get these, get back on this forum and tell us what they were and we might be able to comment on them. One of the more important tests to diagnose Hashimoto's Thyroiditis (the most common cause of hypothyroidism) are the "Thyroid Antibodies Tests". This usually includes the anti-thyroglobulin and anti-thyroperoxidase antibodies. There are also antibodies that help diagnose Graves Disease (Hyperthyroidism) from other types of thyroid disorders but they look at the antibodies in conjunction with thyroid hormone levels. If the hormones are low along with antibodies being elevated, it is certain to be autoimmune hypothyroidism.

Another important thing to remember though, is that with Hashimoto's (autoimmune hypothyroid), you can swing back & forth between hypothyroid & hyperthyroid.

This is because the antibody attack against your thyroid (autoimmune disease), will sometimes actually cause the thyroid to overproduce hormone (intermittent hyperthyroidism) in it's attempt to fight off the attack but it will always return back to a hypothyroid state and will eventually remain so, progressively once enough thyroid tissue has been permanently destroyed by the autoimmune process. This may be why you are having both hyper & hypo symptoms almost simultaneously. I hope this helps, in the mean time, shoot us those lab readings if you can and want to, because most of us out here are very familiar with those due to seeing so many of our own.

QUESTION SIXTY-TWO

Do you know anything about the Evaluation of Thyroid Nodules?

From a forum post I made Re: "The Evaluation of thyroid Nodules".---

Only a very small percent of nodules are cancerous and if they already told you this is not a concern, they are probably certain. They can actually tell what kind of nodule you have by feeling (palpating) it. The size and firmness etc... tells them a lot about the type nodule you have. I think if you go to the new specialist, I would only have it removed if they believe it needs to be. I know it is very hard to accept something being in your body like this, that's causing a problem but I'm not so sure removal of the nodule would stop the autoimmune process. Some researchers believe nodules are simply a symptom of a problem that's deeper inside the thyroid. Try to be patient (easier said than done) because it is good that they are taking time to thoroughly evaluate the best treatment possible for you. In the mean time, shoot us any questions that might come up. We may have helpful opinion or sometimes might not know anything but it always helps to communicate with other fellow-patient sufferers.

QUESTION SIXTY-THREE

Are there Thyroid Antibodies that cause Hypothyroid and Hyperthyroid Symptoms?

From a forum post I made, Re: "Thyroid Antibodies causing Hypothyroid and Hyperthyroid Symptoms".---

First, a person with antibodies can most certainly have thyroid symptoms of both hyperthyroidism and hypothyroidism. If your Dr. doesn't seem to know this, you might think about a new Dr. (but I'm sure he/she does). Your description of symptoms, including the eye irritation are classic for thyroid disorder. It is true that sometimes a Dr.s doesn't know when to treat and is a difficult decision for them when you are totting back and forth between hypo & hyper but this is a common happening when you have Autoimmune Thyroid Disease. In case you haven't been told it is "autoimmune" - that's what it is. If what you have is Hashimoto's Thyroiditis, the hyper times will eventually stop happening because your thyroid will begin to fizzle-out. It actually becomes damaged by the auto-antibodies attacking and it loses its ability to produce adequate levels of thyroid hormone and you'll become permanently "hypothyroid". At that time, they will be able to see this on your hormone blood level tests.

Your TSH which is probably in normal range only for now, will become elevated (the hormone that tries to kick-start your thyroid to produce) and your other thyroid hormones will begin to drop to low levels. Usually, as soon as they see the TSH elevate, they'll treat you with replacement hormone because you also have antibodies.

The hormone will actually shrink any existing goiters or nodules, unless they are the type that need further attention and only your Dr. can determine this.

The medication will also relieve your "hypo" symptoms, although some of us have lingering symptoms such as fatigue and joint aches. Your weight gain and loss also have to do with your condition. You could on the other hand, have Graves' Disease which is also autoimmune but causes only hyperthyroidism and not the hypo symptoms you have along with yours. Graves can be temporary in some cases whereas Hashi's Disease is almost always permanent. With Graves', they sometimes kill off the thyroid gland (oblation) with radio-active iodine because the hyper state causes some people, serious heart and blood pressure problems. Once they kill off a Graves' thyroid, that person has to take thyroid replacement med., just like hypothyroid people do. I've been in your place and needed answers badly so wanted to give you the best summation of thyroid disorders that I could.

QUESTION SIXTY-FOUR

Any Association between Thyroid Disease and Orthostatic Hypotension?

Derived from a forum post I made Re: "Thyroid Disease and Orthostatic Hypotension".---

I have had many times of wondering when these symptoms will get under control! I too had vision problems after getting Hashimoto's thyroiditis. ALSO: That was so interesting your mention of having to stand in one spot until the orthostatic intolerance passed. I've had people see me do this, plus I would steady myself with a hand on the wall and they'd say "what's wrong?" and I'd say "just another dizzy spell from standing up!" This is also called Orthostatic Hypotension" (O.I.) and is a form of "dysautonomia", meaning an imbalance of the automonic nervous system (involuntary nervous system).

This is the part of the N.S. that regulates blood pressure, heart rate etc... Dysautonomia sometimes co-exists with autoimmune diseases. O. I. is not supposed to be harmful or dangerous unless you fall down. They only recommend treatment for it when it is so bad you actually pass out from it. All I know is it sure is a bummer! One last mention of this condition is that researchers have found O.I. to be a common component of both Chronic Fatigue Syndrome and fibromyalgia, which are also now recognized as autoimmune related diseases.

QUESTION SIXTY-FIVE

Should a Treated Hypothyroid Patient be Struggling with Weight Gain?

The post following, was a reply on a thyroid forum I made to a "Treated Hypothyroid Patient Struggling with Weight Gain" and difficulty losing weight.---

You posted a reply to my question about joint aches. I want to reply to yours as well. I'm a male however; I too have an incredible time trying to lose weight since having Hashimoto's/Hypothyroidism. I wanted to do an overall improvement in all areas, including weight, so that I could get ahead of this thing but instead of losing, I've actually gained since being on the medication. I too am not obese but overweight. Please stay encouraged as much as possible, you have friends out here in the same mess you're in. I don't know if it's true because there are so many opinions out there in the medical but some say that once the thyroid completely atrophies (dies off from disease), people then see improvements because the antibody levels then begin to significantly decrease. I hope it's true but regardless, please hang in there and keep researching because you'll find a good nugget once in a while and suggestions that will help. Put them all together at some point and we might have a completed puzzle.

QUESTION SIXTY-SIX

Are there some Uninformed Doctors Treating Thyroid Diseases?

The following is derived from a thyroid support forum post I made in the year 2005 regarding "Uninformed Doctors Treating Thyroid Diseases".---

The more I read others comments, the more amazed I become! I too am terribly frustrated with Doctors (it took me five to get diagnosed). They are overbooked and burned-out and worse than that, they are often totally lacking compassion. I too was diagnosed as a mental case at first and placed on an antidepressant, Xanax and a beta-blocker. These made my untreated thyroid much worse! Some people have not yet understood that most Dr,s today are very uninformed about thyroid disorder for example, you'll hear a Dr. say: "Only a TSH test is necessary to diagnose thyroid imbalance." What's strange about that opinion is the fact that Graves Disease and Hashimoto's thyroiditis both can manifest as "normal TSH" with the actual thyroid hormones being affected independently of the TSH level. ALSO, a person can have symptoms even with all hormones in normal range, if antibody levels remain high because and I quote from many reputable sites; "High antibody levels will cause reduced ability for thyroid hormones to bind to receptors, resulting in hypothyroid symptoms even while levels are in normal range".

WE PATIENTS should not have to do Dr.s jobs! But since this uninformed trend is going on with Dr.s, we better keep researching and sharing research with one another.

QUESTION SIXTY-SEVEN

Can Joint Pain occur with Treated Hypothyroidism?

Article derived from a forum post I made in year 2005, regarding "Joint Pain with Treated Hypothyroidism".---

Thanks, so much ladies for your input, that is truly amazing and I have a feeling it is a common problem with Hashimoto's thyroiditis sufferers. You mentioned joint aches worse with the thyroid hormone replacement medication. Strange you should say that, I often comment to my wife, that my joint aches became much worse with the medication and she remembers this too. Back when I had been on medication only a few months, I got discouraged and so I did a search, using key words "reasons thyroid replacement medication may have adverse effects", or something to that effect and it took me to sights stating "untreated adrenal cortical insufficiency may become worse after starting thyroid medication", in fact ALL BRANDS of thyroid medication have this warning in their literature. So, I searched "symptoms of adrenal insufficiency" and there listed, were the same symptoms for hypothyroid, including fatigue (Which I also still have - do you?), joint pain etc...

This prompted me to order a home Stress Hormone Test from GSMDL, Inc. and over the past year, I have done 4 of these and each time, my cortisol (the major stress hormone) was low normal, borderline low and even clinically low on one of them.

I've also found sites stating that 25% of Hashimoto's patients develop other problems, such as adrenal insufficiency, anemia (I was borderline) and diabetes (borderline on this too). It's funny how the typical Dr. will not tell you these things. Have you ladies read Mary Shomon's book "Living Well with Autoimmune Disease"? I highly recommend it if not. Mary relates experiencing a time of unrelieved symptoms in her book even while on thyroid replacement (she has Hashi's) so I knew I related well to her problem but I wanted to hear from others on this too.

QUESTION SIXTY-EIGHT

Can you share Symptom Problems you experienced with Hypothyroid Treatment?

The following article is derived from a post I made on a thyroid patient support forum in 2005. The post reveals the type "Symptom Problems I Experienced with my Hypothyroid Treatment".---

I'm an age-42 man with Hashimoto's thyroiditis and was wondering if any of you out there with the same, have joint pain even though on medication? I have already been tested for RA Factor, Uric Acid, ANA, ESR possibilities but all were negative.

After being on thyroid med. for two years and getting my TSH in good range "1.0" and my other thyroid hormones in the upper half of the ranges, I asked for the antibodies tests because none of the five Dr.s I've had to go to get proper treatment, would suggest one. My Anti-thyroglobulin ABs were "537" (normal being <40) and my Anti-Peroxidase ABs were "84" (normal being <35).

When I originally was diagnoses hypo, my TSH was "8.3" (high) and the other abnormal was a T-3 Uptake, flagged "low". Other than this, labs were in lower half of normal ranges. The Dr.s claimed this was only "sub-clinical Hypothyroidism" however; this part I know now is BALONEY!

With Hashmoto's, TSH and other levels can fluctuate! ANYWAY, to sum up my question, do you guys/gals believe HIGHANTIBODY LEVELS, can perpetuate symptoms, even while on thyroid replacement? AND, do any of you have joint pain even on treatment? My joint pain is almost all upper body, cervical spine, shoulders and collar bones but occasionally my feet ache in the arches too.

QUESTION SIXTY-NINE

Natural Supplements for Autoimmune Hypothyroidism?

There are natural ways to compliment or what you might call "supplementing" your hypothyroid therapy but none of these are a substitute for thyroid hormone replacement therapy. For example, a healthy diet, exercise and healthy supplements (i.e. vitamins and safe well-researched herbals containing no-iodine) can help, being careful to take those that contain calcium or iron, about six hours apart from thyroid hormone dose. I also believe-in running any supplements past a person's treating doctor, to help determine their safety.

As far as something that can substitute thyroid hormone replacement, there simply is nothing that can do this because the body absolutely requires it. It is also important that you are assured by your doctor that your treatment has been best-possible optimized. He can do this by going over your follow-up blood retests showing where your thyroid hormone levels are. There are medical studies published by the U.S. NIV (PubMed) stating that "selenium" supplementation can reduce antibody levels and activity (i.e. inflammation and selling) in cases of autoimmune hypothyroidism.

Autoimmunity of any kind is a strange phenomenon that medical research is trying to understand more as they conduct further research. Some sources state that autoimmunity is caused by an overactive immune system.

This quote: "People with lupus have an overactive immune system." from MedicineNet.com - By the site Medical Editor: William C. Shiel Jr., MD, FACP, FACR is an example of this opinion.

I also feel in some people, diseases of autoimmunity can point-to immune deficiency because I for example have autoimmune thyroid disease - Hashimoto's thyroiditis but I also have immune deficiency in other areas. I have CFS co-morbid to thyroid autoimmunity and mild asthma which both point-to immune deficiency. It's almost as if in some patients, their immune system contradicts itself (overactive and under active simultaneously) and is why it's so important to have a good doctor to evaluate what's needed in each autoimmune disease patient.

QUESTION SEVENTY

Can TSH at "7.0" Represent Hypothyroidism?

Many blood testing labs are now setting their high-normal cut-off value for TSH at about 4.5, so a reading of 7.0 is elevated. TSH rises above normal with hypothyroidism (under active thyroid). If your thyroid hormone levels are not falling below normal at the same time TSH is rising, you may only have sub-clinical hypothyroidism but only your doctor can tell you for sure. Regardless, if you need treated; it simply requires that your doctor prescribe a daily dose of a thyroid hormone replacement drug. Over time, the dose will correct your low metabolism by getting your thyroid hormones back to euthroid level (normal).

Hypothyroidism can develop before the T3 and/or T4 fall below normal values. Some people see TSH rise to between 10.0 and 15.0 and thyroid hormones are still within normal range. A "7.0" TSH is elevated according to all lab ranges for it that I have seen because highest normal averages about "5.0" at many labs but can be as high as 6.0 at a few of them. Some labs place highest-normal TSH at 4.0 and some experts even believe readings above 3.0 indicate developing hypothyroidism. In my opinion a 7.0 reading merits follow up every few months by repeat blood testing despite normal T3 and T4 levels.

QUESTION SEVENTY-ONE

What is the Goal of Thyroid Hormone Replacement?

The goal of thyroid hormone replacement is to suppress the TSH level (pituitary hormone) and to elevate the T4 and T3 to mid-range or above. A blood TSH level over "10.0" indicates overt (full blown) hypothyroidism. TSH elevates with hypothyroidism, while the thyroid hormones (T4 & T3) decrease to abnormally low levels.

The average normal value at blood testing labs for TSH is 0.4 to 4.5 and your thyroid dose will need to get your TSH back down into this normal values range. Some doctors have a goal of suppressing TSH down to between "1.0 and 2.0" to successfully resolve hypothyroid symptoms of fatigue, weight gain, dry skin, constipation, etc...

Thyroid hormone replacement medications are designed to replace the low level no longer being supplied by the thyroid gland or "hypothyroidism" (under active). This condition causes a slowing of the metabolism which means fuels coming into the body (i.e. food and oxygen) are burned/used at a slower rate. By administering thyroid hormone therapy - dosed to a proper level, the metabolism is brought back up to normal speed.

If once a proper dose level is reached and even more hormone is added (unnecessary dose increase - over treatment) the metabolism then becomes abnormally sped-up. This would be referred to as dose induced "thyrotoxicity" (hyperthyroidism-overactive).

354

An overactive thyroid gland or thyrotoxicity from whatever cause (i.e. Graves' disease, thyroid hormone drug, hot nodules in the thyroid gland) will typically cause weight loss. One reason for this is because food passes through the body too quickly for nutrients to be absorbed or for fat to be stored in the body. This is also why diarrhea is a common symptom listed for hyperthyroidism.

QUESTION SEVENTY-TWO

Can Goiter cause Thyroid Swelling on One Side?

Your isthmus (middle portion of the thyroid) is centered in the gland and the two lobes (one on each side) extend upward and are attached to the Adams apple via connecting cartilage (the Adams apple itself is cartilage). It is a butterfly-shaped gland, located just below the Adams apple in the front-middle of the neck.

When a goiter (swelling) begins, it can affect only one lobe and a lobe can be affected by a "thyroid nodule" causing it to protrude as well. If both goiter and nodule are present, they refer to it as a "nodular goiter".

Your doctor can palpate your gland (feel with fingertips) to see if he detects a nodule and whether if feels firm or not. From there he would likely order a thyroid ultrasound and/or a thyroid uptake scan (radioactive iodine dose, followed by radiological imaging).

If a thyroid nodule if found and is of a large size or it appears solid, a thyroid tissue biopsy might follow or what is also referred to as a "Fine Needle Aspiration" to make sure no cancer cells are present.

If no nodules are found, you may simply be experiencing thyroid autoimmunity with resulting inflammation which will eventually lead to hypothyroidism (low functioning) and the goiter may shrink once you're placed on thyroid hormone replacement - once needed.

356

If you have a mild, temporary goiter which can occur with respiratory viruses, it will resolve over a few weeks time. Your doctor can better determine the cause of the swollen thyroid lobe or even determine that the swelling is not in your thyroid but rather in a lymph node located near the thyroid gland.

QUESTION SEVENTY-THREE

Why Would TSH be Low but Throxine Normal?

This question I respond-to following below, was asked by someone who had a low TSH blood result ("0.287") but a normal T4 (thyroxine level:

A result on TSH of 0.287 is only very slightly below the lowest-normal cut-off value of "0.3". This type result would merit follow up, to make sure it is not continuing to drop because a flagged-low TSH usually represents hyperthyroidism (overactive thyroid). If a lab has "0.25" as the low normal reference range, yours would still be within normal but being near borderline, would still merit a repeat blood test within a few months to see if it has dropped further. Testing both the T3 and T4 thyroid hormone levels might be wise as well and tests for thyroid antibodies - the immune cells that cause autoimmune thyroid disease.

Some people have TSH levels that do not accurately reflect their thyroid hormone levels and I'm one of them. As a treated hypothyroid patient (under active thyroid gland), my TSH has to be suppressed to below normal to get my thyroxine (T4) and my T3 levels up to at least mid-range. TSH normally elevates with hypothyroidism and usually goes low with hyperthyroidism (overactive).

Another possibility is that you have a pituitary gland problem - the one that sends TSH to the thyroid, causing it to release proper amounts of hormone. If there is a small tumor in the pituitary it can cause it to be sluggish in sending enough TSH, which is referred-to as "hypopituitarism".

If this is the case, your thyroxine may have been normal-range but in the "low-normal". Over time, if it is your pituitary failing to send adequate amounts of TSH to stimulate the thyroid gland, you'll eventually develop "Central Hypothyroidism" (failure of the central command - brain center).

The third possibility is that you are very early into the onset of hyperthyroidism and your TSH is starting to go lower as your thyroxine level rises. Over time, the thyroxine will go outside of the normal values (flagged high) if this is the case. Graves' disease is the most common cause of hyperthyroidism, so you may need to be tested for "thyroid antibodies" that cause the disease - referred to as "Thyroid Stimulating Immunoglobulin".In my opinion your TSH and thyroxine levels merit follow up blood retesting as well within two or three months, so would discuss this with your doctor.

QUESTION SEVENTY-FOUR

Can Elevated Thyroid Hormone Levels cause Anxiety?

Anxiety, nervousness and panic attacks are listed commonly for hyperthyroid conditions (overactive thyroid), including Graves' disease (autoimmune caused) and a condition called "Hashitoxicosis" which can occur, just before a person begins to experience hypothyroidism (under active thyroid).

When a goiter (thyroid swelling) occurs with hyperthyroidism, it is called a "toxic diffuse goiter" and if small tumor-like growths develop in the gland, that causes it to produce excessive amounts of hormone, it is called a "hot nodule". Someone being treated for hypothyroidism with thyroid hormone replacement can develop anxiety symptoms as well if their dose is too high, which is called "thyrotoxicity".

All of these hyperthyroid conditions have potential to cause anxiety symptoms and if you do a search using "hyperthyroid symptoms" as a term with a search engine, this will come up often as part of the symptom-complex.

Yes, thyroid imbalance can most definitely manifest with anxiety symptoms, among others.

QUESTION SEVENTY-FIVE

Can Hyperthyroidism be resolved with Drug Treatment Only?

The answer that follows below, was to a question posted to me by a hyperthyroid patient who was treated with an anti-thyroid drug only (NeoMercazole) and afterward they were placed on thyroid hormone replacement (Eltroxin) for hypothyroidism. It is actually rare for hyperthyroid cases to not require destruction or removal of the thyroid gland and is one of several points I made in my comments to them that follow. ---

NeoMercazole is an antithyroid medication that slows thyroid hormone production in an overactive gland. With your hyperthyroidism resolving with this medication and not also requiring thyroid removal, it may have been a rare case in which Graves' disease (autoimmune caused hyperthyroidism) resolved without further treatment. It may also be that your case was actually that of Hashimoto's thyroiditis(autoimmune caused hypothyroidism) which can first present with a phase of hyperthyroidism – "Hashitoxicosis".

Your doctor could order tests for Anti-TPO and anti-TG antibodies and if one or both are positive, Hashimoto's would be a strong possibility. A tissue biopsy called an "FNA" (Fine Needle Aspiration) and a thyroid ultrasound would help confirm this as well, plus the latter one can help detect whether any thyroid nodules are present. The type called "hot nodules" can also be a cause of hyperthyroidism.

Eltroxin is a thyroid hormone replacement drug and many Thyroid Specialists and Endocrinologists suggest getting the TSH level (a blood hormone level most often used to monitor thyroid hormone replacement) suppressed down to between "1.0 and 2.0" to better optimized relief of hypothyroid symptoms (like fatigue). Some use "1.0" as their target treatment goal. These are things you might consider discussing with your doctor, to better understand your case.

QUESTION SEVENTY-SIX

Do Thyroid Antibodies Continue with Hypothyroid Therapy?

Hashimoto's is a lifelong autoimmune thyroiditis and the resulting hypothyroidism it causes requires permanent treatment as well. Some people diagnosed with underactive thyroid glands are not afterward tested for causes of it but the most common cause in industrialized countries like the UK and US is Hashimoto's. Treating doctors vary in how often they blood retest their hypothyroid patients, to see how thyroid hormone replacement is going.

If retests are only done once-yearly or even twice, the TSH level (likely the one that was elevated when you were tested) can go up, indicating a need for a higher replacement dose to suppress the TSH level back down into the normal range.

As far as thyroid antibody levels go, these will fluctuate in autoimmune thyroiditis patients, throughout their lives and doesn't usually represent how well the hypothyroidism is treated. Some patients see them lower with hormone therapy but this is not always true.

What I describe above has been the case with my treatment as a hypothyroid patient with Hashimoto's (thyroid antibodies are sometimes elevated, even with optimal treatment) and is how many medical sources also explain it.

Thyroid diseases run in families and some members may see hyperthyroidism develop from Graves' disease and from the antibodies that contribute to it (thyroid stimulating immunoglobulin "TSI"). Others have the antibodies that contribute to Hashimoto's being the "anti-thyroidperoxidase" (TPO) and the "anti-thyroglobulin" (TG). You might consider asking your doctor to go over your blood test results with you, to help you better understand these issues.

QUESTION SEVENTY-SEVEN

Is Blood Testing - A Doctor's Greatest Diagnostic Tool?

When I saw the first doctor for my thyroid symptoms, she diagnosed me with emotional only problems - "Generalized Anxiety Disorder". What puzzled me however was the fact that my very dry skin and joint/muscle aches that I complained of would also be considered emotional-only symptoms. I saw a different doctor to have blood tests ordered and my thyroid disease (hypothyroidism caused by Hashimoto's thyroiditis) was found.

I feel that due to doctors having problems with less-than detailed patients, who sometimes fail to fully relate their symptoms and doctors who may be overbooked and unable to spend as much time as needed with patients on certain days, blood testing should be resorted-to often. It is so incredibly diagnostic and only requires a stroke-of-the-pen to get them ordered. I agree with the opinion that has been stated by medical sources, that lifetime viruses, allergens and environmental toxins can all cause our immune systems to go haywire over time and lots of medical research studies back this up. I have written on the fact that when a virus cannot be fully eradicated by the immune system, it may then resort to attacking the tissues in the body that contain them.

For these reasons, blood testing should be ordered for symptomatic patients who may have problems going on in their bodies that may not otherwise be diagnosed.

QUESTION SEVENTY-EIGHT

What Importance is there in Thyroid Antibodies Blood Tests?

In my lay opinion, but one that is based on lots of research on medical research sites and correspondence with literally 1,000s of fellow thyroid patients since year-2003, if thyroid disease runs in a family, "thyroid antibodies" test should also be tested for when blood labs are being done. These are the "anti-throidperoxidase" (TPO) and the "anti-thyroglobulin" (TG) and if either or both are positive, autoimmune thyroid disease is present regardless of thyroid hormone levels.

I have friends with Hashimoto's thyroiditis whose thyroid hormones were within normal range but their TPO antibody levels tested in the 1,000s. In some cases their doctors started them on thyroid hormone replacement therapy, which in some cases can slow down thyroid autoimmunity and because some of them had mild to moderate goiters (thyroid gland swelling).

In my case for example - when I was diagnosed with hypothyroidism, my TSH was only moderately elevated @ "8.3" (normal range 0.4 to 4.5) and by thyroid hormones were only at mid-range or slightly below. At the same time my TG antibodies were @ "537" (range <40) so were almost 500 points above normal. My TPO antibodies were @ "120" (range <35). I was experiencing hypothyroid symptoms despite normal-range thyroid hormones. Your thyroid ABs may be negative but testing them will help rule out thyroid disease or confirm its presence.

QUESTION SEVENTY-NINE

Is My Hashimoto's Thyroiditis caused by Mononucleosis?

I too have Hashimoto's and treated for the hypothyroidism that resulted from it. I had mononucleosis at about age 10 and it was a severe case, keeping me out of school for six weeks. At age 40, both the thyroid disease and CFS manifested and my belief is that these can be traced-back to my bout of mono from the EBV virus.

When I was tested for EBV antibodies a few years ago, at my request, due to my thyroid treatment not alleviating the CFS symptoms, my result was "218" - the normal range being <20 (20 and above being positive). While 80% or more of the population has the EBV in their system, CFS and other autoimmune disease patients, including those with MS, often have very high titers of EBV antibodies (like mine).

This means the virus can remain in a highly replicated state in susceptible individuals (post viral illness) and medical research associates high titers with development of certain types of diseases and syndromes like CFS. This fact is also recognized by the U.S. National Institutes of Health.

QUESTION EIGHTY

Is Hypothyroid Treatment Available for Heart Patients?

Thyroid disease medical resources state that people being treated for heart conditions are usually replaced on thyroid hormone to correct their low thyroid hormone levels by suppressing the TSH level back down into the higher normal values range. TSH elevates with hypothyroidism and if the highest normal value for it at a blood testing lab is about 4.5 for example, the thyroid dose might only be adjusted to suppress the TSH no lower than 3.0 or 4.0.

It depends on how severe your doctor determines your heart condition to be and how well controlled it is on your current treatments. Increasing the metabolism in the body via thyroid hormone can place added stress on the heart and is why it may be less-optimized in a heart patient than it would be in a patient with no cardiac issues.

QUESTION EIGHTY-ONE

What are the Pros and Cons of RAI Thyroid Gland Ablation?

After corresponding with literally 1,000s of thyroid patients since, year-2003, much of this being when I moderated patient-forums, lots of stories were related to me by patients who underwent RAI ablation, who had adverse reactions to it. Some saw a worsening of their thyroid eye disease for example, after weeks post-procedure. Others had successful ablations with no complications. This is why patients referred for the treatment should be thoroughly informed about risks and given the option of surgical thyroidectomy as an alternative choice.

Thyroidectomies also have risks, such as inadvertent damage or removal of parathyroid glands but if a patient has difficult-to-treat hyperthyroidism, they must undergo one or the other (RAI ablation or surgical removal) because if severe hyperthyroidism is allowed to continue, heart problems and severe bone loss can occur. These risks are also why I personally believe patients should first have drug treatment attempted (i.e. anti-thyroid and/or beta-blocker drugs) before thyroid-removal options are offered. If these are not successful, then a choice has to me made between these other two options. Lots of endocrinologists and thyroid specializing MDs agree with this opinion.

It is difficult if not impossible to fully cover a procedure like RAI in a single article and by attempting to do so, articles become too lengthy, so that readers seeking general info will bypass them.

What one seeking information on this subject should consider doing, is writing down the specific areas of information you are seeking in regard to RAI and discuss those with your doctor or post them on a doctor-moderated forum, that has questions answered by a board certified endocrinologist or thyroid-specializing MD of some type.

QUESTION EIGHTY-TWO

Can Hashimoto's Thyroiditis go into Remission?

It is extremely rare for Hashimoto's autoimmune thyroiditis to go into remission and is in most cases, a life-long disease. The treatment is for the hypothyroidism it causes, once the antibodies that cause the disease have done damage to the thyroid gland and it no longer produces enough hormone. Replacement thyroid hormone drugs are the treatment and it is monitored via follow-up blood tests 1 to 3 times yearly. Some patients do not see complete relief of symptoms and sometimes, there is no explanation as to why this happens but may be the disease aspect rather than imbalanced hormones that contribute to ongoing symptoms.

Getting a replacement hormone dose best-optimized by the treating doctor is all that can be done. If one is taking a T4-only replacement hormone, they might consider asking their doctor to place them on a trial of combination T4 and T3 which gives better symptom relief to some patients and while not true in all cases, might be worth a trial if a doctor is willing. If other causes of symptoms are suspected, blood tests should be ordered to rule these out or to confirm them as co morbid conditions. This can be things like anemia, vitamin deficiencies, blood glucose imbalances and sex or adrenal hormone imbalances. Thyroid disease places these conditions at slightly higher risk for developing than in the general public, according to some medical research studies.

QUESTION EIGHTY-THREE

Should there be A Lowered Upper-Limit TSH Normal Values Range?

The NACB and other medical groups have suggested the 2.5 upper limit cut off for blood TSH levels because if I remember correctly, they have found that 95% of the healthy population has a TSH normal value that is below 2.5, which would mean that levels at 2.5 and above can indicate developing hypothyroidism. One medical research group that has published a study in regard to this suggested revision in the normal range, is the Journal of Clinical Endocrinology & Metabolism - the link to it is here: http://jcem.endojournals.org/cgi/content/full/92/12/4560

This is an even lower upper limit than that suggested by the AACE and would likely detect more borderline and early onset cases as these medical groups are pointing out. If not for the AACE starting the ball rolling, labs would all likely still have the 5.0 and 6.0 upper-limit TSH value ranges.

QUESTION EIGHTY-FOUR

Could my Trembling Hands Indicate a Thyroid Problem?

An overactive thyroid gland (hyperthyroidism) can cause tremor, especially in the hands. A simple blood test called "TSH" (Thyroid Stimulating Hormone) can help to determine if you've developed a hyperthyroid disorder. The TSH, which comes from the pituitary gland, rather than from the thyroid gland, begins to drop to low-normal, and below-normal levels with the onset of hyperthyroidism. If you have the test ordered by your Doc and it's low or borderline-low, you could then have the actual thyroid hormones testes (T3 and T4) to see how severe the hyperthyroidism is. With the thyroid hormones, they do the opposite of TSH and elevate when the thyroid is overactive. If hyperthyroidism is confirmed, a test for "thyroid antibodies" might also be needed, which are the cells from the immune system that attach to the thyroid gland, causing it to over-produce hormones. These are called "thyroid stimulating immunoglobulin" (TSI). If these are positive, Graves' disease (autoimmune cause) would likely be the diagnosis.

If you have hyperthyroidism there are treatments to slow the thyroid gland down and to treat symptoms of sped-up metabolism and the associated anxiety, nervousness and trembling.

Other than these suggestions, I would consider whether you have been taking any new supplements or drugs that might have a stimulating effect on your system, since this can be a cause of hand tremors as well.

QUESTION EIGHTY-FIVE
What Thyroid Test Result Indicates Hypothyroidism when Elevated?

That would be the TSH level (Thyroid Stimulating Hormone) and it is a pituitary hormone rather than a thyroid one but is very accurate and sensitive in reflecting how well the thyroid gland is functioning. It will actually become abnormal in early-onset thyroid disease cases, even before the thyroid hormones (T4 and T3) fall outside of normal range.

TSH begins to rise when the thyroid gland begins under functioning (hypothyroidism). Many blood testing labs have a normal-values range that is approximately from "0.5 to 5.0", so that anything above 5.0 is indicative of a hypothyroid condition.

Some thyroid specializing MDs and endocrinologists believe that a TSH at 10.0 and above, reveals "overt" hypothyroidism (full blown), regardless of where the T4 and/or T3 levels are at. With a TSH of "65" as yours is, your T4 and T3 are likely below normal and you are in need of thyroid hormone replacement therapy to correct the hypothyroidism. The treatment is simple and consists of taking a pill containing the proper dose-level of thyroid hormone to correct your low levels of them.

QUESTION EIGHTY-SIX

Why Do Treated Hypothyroid Patients have Weight Loss Difficulties?

I'm a male hypothyroid patient, so can give you an answer from personal experience. Also, I've know Mary Shomon for years, from the about.com thyroid disease site (great source of information) and I have in fact written reviews for her books, that she has sent me copies of, including "The Thyroid Diet".

I recommend you get a copy of that book, which you can find on a number of sources, including Amazon by doing a search using the title.

I too have had difficulty with weight loss since the onset of thyroid disease (hypothyroidism, caused by Hashimoto's thyroiditis). I am not terribly overweight but enough-so, that it places me at higher risk for things like diabetes.

I don't mind relating my weight - which is 240lb at 6ft tall. I carry mine well because it evenly gains in my body, rather than just around my middle but I don't like the negative effect it has on my energy levels, so I am working hard on losing some pounds.

With us thyroid patients it just simply takes more effort to lose weight and keep it off, than it does for the healthy public. My suspicion is that even treated hypothyroidism, still adversely affects bodily metabolism, subtly but enough-so, as to make it difficult to keep extra pounds off.

You can probably find Mary's dieting guidelines in-summation at her about.com or her thyroid-info.com site, in addition to her in-print book. You will increase your odds in successful weight loss and in maintaining it, if you seriously implement those as part of your treatment regimen. We must do our part, in addition to what our doctor is doing for us (be proactive).

Best wishes with it, from a fellow-patient who is rooting for you!

QUESTION EIGHTY-SEVEN

What are some of the Main Causes of Hypothyroidism?

Hypothyroidism can be caused by a number of things but in the more industrialized countries, the cause is "thyroid autoimmunity", also called "autoimmune thyroiditis" and "Hashimoto's disease". It is a process in which the thyroid gland becomes under active after being relentlessly attacked by auto-antibodies sent from the immune system that mistakenly identify it as an intruder, as it would allergens, bacteria and viruses. Once enough thyroid cells are damaged by these antibodies over time, hypothyroidism sets in.

In the less industrialized countries, where iodine rich foods are lacking or they do not have access to iodized sale, "iodine deficiency hypothyroidism" can be the cause. Other causes are things like a failure in the brain glands that regulate thyroid function (master-gland endocrine failure) which is called "central hypothyroidism". Women can develop a temporary form of thyroiditis when pregnant, that leaves them hypothyroid afterward, called "postpartum hypothyroidism" which can in some cases be temporary and other times permanent, needing lifelong treatment.

Some people are born with insufficient thyroid glands (small or partially missing) and as they enter their teens or adult years, their thyroid hormone levels become inadequate. This is referred to as "congenital hypothyroidism" and in some cases is diagnosed at birth and treated, with no negative consequences as the child develops.

People, who experience severe throat injuries, such as in car accidents, can damage their thyroid glands to the extent that they become under active and lastly, a person can experience hypothyroidism following exposure to chemicals or drugs that adversely affect the thyroid gland, called "chemical hypothyroidism". Lots of Russian people experienced hypothyroidism following the Chernobyl nuclear power plant accident in 1986, in which nuclear fallout affected their thyroid glands in years following, causing them to become under active.

At the basic level, an under active thyroid simply means one that is not producing enough hormone to properly regulate bodily metabolism.

(END - SECTION SEVEN)

THE END

www.ingramcontent.com/pod-product-compliance
Lightning Source LLC
Chambersburg PA
CBHW060233290526
45789CB00001B/25